BAREFOOT SHIATSU

BAREFOOT
SHIATSU

Shizuko Yamamoto

Japan Publications, Inc.

© 1979 by Japan Publications, Inc.

Published by
JAPAN PUBLICATIONS, INC., Tokyo, Japan

Distributors:
UNITED STATES: *Kodansha International/USA, Ltd., through Harper & Row, Publishers, Inc., 10 East 53rd Street, New York, New York 10022.* SOUTH AMERICA: *Harper & Row, Publishers, Inc., International Department.* CANADA: *Fitzhenry & Whiteside Ltd., 150 Lesmill Road, Don Mills, Ontario M3B 2T6.* MEXICO AND CENTRAL AMERICA: *HARLA S. A. de C. V., Apartado 30–546, Mexico 4, D. F.* BRITISH ISLES: *International Book Distributors Ltd., 66 Wood Lane End, Hemel Hempstead, Herts HPZ 4RG.* EUROPEAN CONTINENT: *Boxer books, Inc., Limmatstrasse 111, 8031 Zurich.* AUSTRALIA AND NEW ZEALAND: *Book Wise (Australia) Pty. Ltd., 104–8 Sussex Street, Sydney 2000.* THE FAR EAST AND JAPAN: *Japan Publications Trading Co., Ltd., 1–2–1, Sarugaku-cho, Chiyoda-ku, Tokyo 101.*

First edition: March 1979
Second printing: February 1981

ISBN 0–87040–439–3

Printed in U.S.A.

Dedication

With deepest thanks to my parents who gave me the chance to live in this world, to George and Lima Ohsawa for the opportunities they opened for me, and to the many friends in both the East and the West who have helped and encouraged me, I dedicate this book.

Foreword

I met Shizuko Yamamoto, the author of this book, upon her arrival from Japan in June 1965, which was her first visit to the United States. Already at that time, the name of Shizuko Yamamoto was well-known among the circle of Macrobiotic people in Japan, especially around Tokyo.

Like myself, she had passed through the experience of hardship during World War II, in which millions of precious human lives and hundreds of traditional cities were destroyed. Undoubtedly, through the misery and confusion of warfare, Shizuko Yamamoto developed her deep concern for human affairs, and for the establishment of a better society and a peaceful world. As everyone can easily see when they meet her, Shizuko Yamamoto radiates the light of love and sympathy toward people.

During the difficult post-war period, Shizuko Yamamoto learned from several masters of oriental physio-therapeutic arts. Through this, together with her unique native ability, she gained her profound understanding of human nature and way of life in general. Especially during this period, she encountered the teaching of the Macrobiotic Way of Life, which encompasses the eternal, universal order and dietary approach as the basis of human happiness. George Ohsawa (Yukikazu Sakurazawa) and Lima Ohsawa, as well as many other people in the Macrobiotic and oriental medical field around that time, enriched her development. Among these were Master Seiya Noguchi, and Master Masahiro Oki.

Upon her arrival in America, however, she continued her studies and development on her own. She lived with our family in Boston for a short time before proceeding to her major residence in New York City. In this great populated city of modern civilization, she has acted as one of the central figures in enlightening people through her charming personality, enriched experience, and her unique skills in the art of physiotherapy, centering around the traditional way of massage. During these years she has received more than 20,000 visitors who sought her advice on their physical and mental problems. To each of these visitors she gave understanding, advice, and encouragement, teaching a great number the invaluable benefits of the art of physical-mental adjustment.

Not only has she given such guidance to individuals, but she has also taught her arts of massage, theory, and practice to some thousands of people in the many discussions, meetings, lectures, and seminars in which she has participated. I myself have taught oriental arts of massage and other physiotherapies in the New England area since 1968, but since Shizuko Yamamoto joined us I have actively recommended her way of treatment because her arts have wide appeal not only for professionals but for the lay person's use with friends and families.

Shizuko Yamamoto has taught throughout the United States, in such cities as New York, Boston, Philadelphia, Washington, D.C., Miami, Chicago, Los Angeles, San Francisco, and Seattle. Many of these classes were sponsored by the East West Foundation, which is an educational-cultural organization for the promotion of a better understanding of East and West and for the pursuit of realizing One Peaceful World through the Macrobiotic principle—that is, the understanding of the Order of the Universe. Many other organizations, associations, and educational institutions have also sponsored her teaching, however, and as a result many thousands of people are now practicing the art of massage for their own health as well as for others.

For the past two years, Shizuko Yamamoto has begun visiting Europe as well, teaching and guiding people in such countries as England, Holland, Belgium, France, Switzerland, Italy, Portugal, and Spain. She continues to be a central figure in the East West Macrobiotic Center in New York, devoting her life to achieving better relations between different cultures in order to achieve a better society through better health.

I am very pleased that she has written *Barefoot Shiatsu*, and I recommend it highly to all professional people, including those in the medical, psychological, and physiotherapeutic fields, as well as to all people who are interested in the natural arts of healing. I also recommend this book to all single and family people who will be able to practice upon themselves and their family members to preserve an energetic daily life.

All departments of oriental medicine—such as acupuncture, moxibustion, herbal medicine, various physiotherapies, and the Macrobiotic Way of Life—are based upon the understanding of the Order of the Universe, the principle of change of energies and vibrations. So also is the art of Shizuko Yamamoto based upon the principle of yin and yang, the everlasting law of change.

This law of change is a concept that is fundamental to various ancient cultures, their customs, manners, and way of life, and has been interpreted at the very foundation of Shintoism, Confucianism, Taoism, Vedantic philosophy, Judaism, and original Christianity. The recovery of the understanding of this law of change is the most important requirement for this present world to unify all the conflicting sciences, ideologies, thoughts, arts, and cultures. In order to establish world peace and human happiness, it is essential that these principles of the

Order of the Universe are again clearly understood by all people, and as they apply to such various fields as chemistry, physics, biology, astronomy, agriculture, food processing, economics, politics, religion, education, and all other emotional, intellectual manifestations.

The work of Shizuko Yamamoto successfully manifests these principles in her arts and techniques. Her way does not stay only in the solution to the problem of health, therefore, but can be extended toward the establishment of a peaceful society and world. I hope everyone will read and master *Barefoot Shiatsu*.

October 1978

MICHIO KUSHI
Brookline, Massachusetts

Preface

I was born at a time when many Japanese became interested in the ways of the West. At that time, anything that was new to Japan was seen as desirable, and more traditional Japanese ways were not as popular. As a consequence, I received a western type of education, and was raised on a typically western diet of meat, sugar and rich foods. I had a very happy youth. At that time I had complete confidence in my health and felt myself to be physically and spiritually sound. Of course, at that time I thought of mind and body as separate. I felt that even if I had some sort of bodily sickness, I could still become very spiritual. And then, suddenly overnight, I lost the sight in my right eye.

In the course of the next three years, I went to many doctors and underwent many treatments. I took all sorts of medications and had twelve eye operations, but to no avail. During this time, I had few other activities. My only pleasures were to play the piano, listen to music and to cook and eat delicious food. I could do little else. Soon my body became heavier and heavier. My strength declined to the point where even the simplest of exercises was tiresome to me. I began to have stiff shoulders, body aches and pains. I could not sleep. My thinking became very negative. I was no longer happy.

During this time I went to a shiatsu therapist and received my first treatment. I began to relax and feel much better, but I realized that if I did not continue to have treatments, I would become uncomfortable again. I did not like the idea of depending upon someone else to make me feel healthy, and I knew, after three long years of difficulties, that my family, friends and doctors were not going to cure me. At about this time, I was introduced to the macrobiotic way of life and yoga exercises, and I began to realize that I myself was responsible for my own well-being. Soon afterward I changed my life-style. I began to eat brown rice and vegetables. I would arise in the early morning to do yoga *asana* and breathing exercises in the fresh air. And in a positive way I began to push myself to do difficult things. Within a month I was much stronger and I began to think more positively about life.

Until that time I had had absolutely no interest in oriental medicine, but now an interest began to grow within me. Soon I started the study of shiatsu, acupuncture, *seitai* (structural realignment) and Chinese medicine. I also began the study of *aikidō*, the Japanese martial art, and learned about the importance of *hara* and the flow of *ki* throughout the body. My thinking became very different.

Over the next several years I studied these things on a more formal basis both at established schools and with private teachers. At this time I was not concerned with getting a degree or certificate, and I had no intention of ever being a massage therapist; I was simply consumed by my interest in oriental healing. Soon afterward I began to treat people by shiatsu and much to my surprise I learned that if my patient felt better from my treatment then I felt good as well. This was a great change from my previous way of thinking; before I never would have imagined that I could have been happy treating others.

As I treated increasingly more people, my technique naturally began to develop through experience. Then, at the suggestion of George Ohsawa I came to the United States in 1965. In the thirteen years since my arrival I have treated more than 20,000 people and I have taught my technique in various places in Europe and the United States.

My way of thinking has changed dramatically since I discovered, and began to practice the macrobiotic way of life. I no longer think of the mind and body as isolated entities. Shiatsu helped me to understand the imbalances in my own body and this enabled me to understand imbalances in others. In my opinion, the practice of shiatsu together with the macrobiotic diet can lead a person to a strong state of good health. With this in mind, I have created this book.

If this is useful as a textbook, or as an aid to someone suffering from a physical or spiritual affliction, then I will be very happy.

I would like to extend my warmest thanks to Patrick and Meredith McCarty who greatly helped in the preparation of this book. They are currently teaching and practicing my techniques and macrobiotic cooking and philosophy in Eureka, California. Special thanks, as well, must be given to Willy Berliner, who edited and reworked the manuscript. Willy is currently director of The Balancing Point in Portsmouth, New Hampshire, a vegetarian-style natural foods cafe and teaching center, and a division of Macro Polo, Inc., a company specializing in the manufacture and sale of tools and natural fiber products.

Contents

Introduction

The art of healing massage is as old as mankind. Instinctively man has touched the ailing parts of his body to alleviate symptoms of pain. Barefoot shiatsu follows this natural movement of self-healing and takes it a step further for it systematically stimulates the receiver of the massage in such a way as to permit his natural healing power to surface and act. Thus the individual is responsible for his own well-being; he is not dependent upon others for the changes in his body.

The attitude of barefoot shiatsu is best understood as the firm and loving guidance of a mother to her children. The mother gives direction to her children, always pointing the way to a happy, healthy life. She knows her children, and her knowledge permits her to guide them. In much the same way, the practitioner of barefoot shiatsu gives a clear direction to the patient. Shiatsu never cures the patient entirely, it simply awakens his own healing power. Ultimately it is the patient who cures himself.

Literally, shiatsu means finger (shi) pressure (atsu), and in general, shiatsu is stimulation of the body with the hands and fingers. Barefoot shiatsu differs in its endeavor to treat and balance the whole person, harmonizing both mind and body. To do this, the practitioner uses his whole body. Wholeness brings wholeness.

Many of the techniques of barefoot shiatsu involve the use of the feet. The foot can be used in as sensitive a manner as the hand. Using the feet allows the practitioner to keep his posture straight which enables him to breathe more deeply. As a consequence he is able to give a deeper, fuller shiatsu without becoming tired.

The art of shiatsu involves much more than the giving of treatment. The practitioner must first of all be very healthy. He must train himself very well. And through this training he will come to understand himself very well. This sort of self-training is not a military system. It is not training from the outside, but from the inside, for true training comes from the self. Discipline is of the utmost importance, for without it the giver of shiatsu can learn little about himself. Discipline leads naturally to health, and the healthy practitioner is best qualified to treat others. A shiatsu given by a weak person does not feel good. It is a waste of time.

Barefoot shiatsu brings tangible benefits to the giver as well as the receiver. Both should have a strong, good feeling. Both must finish with a feeling of satisfaction and well-being. In order for this to happen they must become one; this requires technique and practice.

The giver of shiatsu must have a healthy body, high intelligence and well-developed intuition. He must be strong and should not tire easily. His thinking must be clear and precise, and his movement and actions must spring from a deep sense of intuition. These qualities will not only allow him to give a strong shiatsu, but will also enable him to change his own physical condition from sickness to health.

Barefoot shiatsu has a very broad view. In a very practical sense it helps to bring about world peace for it helps to bring the receiver into harmony with a greater whole. When you fully understand this deeper significance of massage therapy, the quality and results of your personal application will be very effective.

1. Training the Whole Person

As in any other serious activity, in order to perform barefoot shiatsu well, one must cultivate a total attitude. In other words, barefoot shiatsu should not be practiced casually. This practice should be well-integrated with all other aspects of the shiatsu practitioner's life. Thus the giver of treatment must above all be working on his own self-development. Personal training in the practical aspects of daily living is the first step toward this development. Order must be made in his everyday life. Everything that he undertakes should be done well and completely. He should train himself to the extent that he can respond accurately and immediately to common and crisis situations in the family, at work or with his country.

After one has succeeded in understanding the importance of training the whole person and has established his own practice, he is ready to continue with the second part of training, the practical application of barefoot shiatsu techniques. This is discussed in Chapter Three. When he has developed his technique, he must then give away his knowledge and actively work for things outside himself. To aid and treat others is to continue in self-development. This is the distinctive attitude of barefoot shiatsu.

The barefoot shiatsu technique endeavors to treat and balance the person as a whole. Individual symptoms are noted, but the cause of the symptoms and the entire condition of the person are the primary concerns. The patient's view of life, his family relationships, his occupation and his activities are all considered, for all of these aspects combine to make the whole person.

The term "treatment" can be applied in a much wider sense. Our human society is based upon giving to others. Thus it is very natural to treat others. In fact everyday we treat and are treated by other people. If you buy a coffee for a friend, for example you are treating him. In much the same way, anyone can give a shiatsu treatment to another. To give a good, satisfying treatment, however, is sometimes very difficult. To really succeed at changing a patient's condition requires a developed, whole person. It is not enough to have the curiosity and the desire to alter imbalances. One must also practice and develop oneself so that one's response comes naturally and intuitively. The act of continually analyzing and thinking can suppress this native ability to respond. Self-training, however, permits this natural power to surface and guide one's actions.

If one is not happy and healthy, one cannot satisfactorily treat another. To begin with one must establish one's own health. One must also develop one's self through study. Without study one's development stagnates and one remains unhappy.

We can divide our daily life into four activities: thinking, moving, eating, and sleeping. In the case of the shiatsu practitioner, his thinking should be clear, his movement should be direct and smooth, his daily food should be wholesome and his sleep should be sound. To be a whole person, these actions must be accomplished smoothly and harmoniously. If one thinks, moves, eats, and sleeps well, one will be able to keep up with the constant changes that constitute life. This is the secret of happiness.

Breathing

Through our breathing we communicate with the external world and, in a larger sense, with the universe. Breathing is absolutely essential to life. Without breath we cannot live for very long, and if our breathing is incorrect, we shorten our lives. When we are breathing properly, we become unified with the breath of the universe. In this way, correct breathing can lead to a deeper level of health.

What then is breathing? On the cellular level it is an exchange of gases. We inhale air containing oxygen into our lungs where it is exchanged for carbon dioxide. Thus, in our breathing we communicate as well with the vegetable kingdom.

Oxygen is the body's nourishment, carbon dioxide is the body's waste. When the body is lacking in oxygen, various sicknesses may arise, such as cancer, tuberculosis and high blood pressure. Viral infections often occur in the upper part of the lung because it has less activity in comparison to the lower parts of the lung. Insufficient oxygen may also cause malfunctions in the digestive, nervous and endocrine systems. Such malfunctions lead to fatigue and sickness. Regardless of the food a person takes in, if his breathing remains poor, he will be unable to relieve these fatigue symptoms. In many cases, however, if deep breathing is recommended to those suffering from such ailments, recovery comes very quickly.

Long-term muscle tension is one cause of hardening of the arteries and its attendant high blood pressure. With deep breathing, the muscles relax and become softer and the blood pressure decreases; circulation improves and the overall body metabolism increases. Hardening of the arteries most easily affects the heart and kidneys as well as the renal arteries. The hands and feet are also likely to become hardened because of their location at the body's extremities where oxygen is received last.

A lack of oxygen in the body manifests itself with the following symptoms: with 5 percent less oxygen than normal, there will be a feeling of dizziness and sometimes nausea; with 15 percent less oxygen than normal, the person will faint; and with 30 percent less oxygen than normal, the person will die. Thus oxygen is indeed the most important nourishment.

The average person breathes sixteen times per minute. Some people who practice deep breathing, like practitioners of *Pranayama* Yoga, can receive as much as three to five times more oxygen than an ordinary person. With daily practice of such deep breathing techniques, nervous tension slowly lessens and disappears.

To move smoothly and nobly, one must exhale strongly. To increase one's fighting spirit, one must breathe forcefully in and out. In this way, one can consciously increase one's vitality. To control another, simply breathe longer than he does and he will follow you easily.

The science of *Pranayama* is one branch of the Yoga system. *Prana* is the Indian term for *ki* (Japanese), or *chi* (Chinese), and can be roughly translated to mean "breath" or "life force." The practice of *Pranayama* increases one's personal supply of ki. Paradoxically enough, this is done by giving ki away; the more ki a person gives away, the more ki he can receive. In much the same way, when one is treating someone with shiatsu, if one is consciously giving ki, one will receive ample ki in return. In this way, the giver can treat many people without fatigue.

How to Practice

There are many ways of breathing and hundreds of exercises to develop breathing power. The three methods which follow are among the most basic, and are very beneficial in self-training.

(1) Tanden Natural Breathing

Lie down on your back and close your eyes. Place the soles of your feet on the floor and close to your buttocks. The knees are raised and are held together. This position makes the abdomen comfortable and relaxed. Place the hands on the navel and concentrate on the point

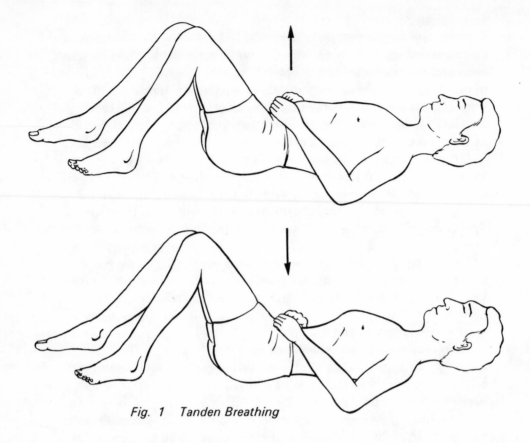

Fig. 1   Tanden Breathing

two-fingers' width below the navel and a little bit to the inside (*tanden*).
Breathe naturally and deeply. You should feel your diaphragm move up
and down. On exhalation contract the anus. Keep your attention on
the point beneath the navel. When 90 percent of the breath has been
released, allow inhalation to come about naturally. Without stopping,
repeat this cycle. On both inhalation and exhalation you may count
slowly—1, 2, 3, 4, 5. Breathe slowly and deeply. Concentrate on the *hara*.

This type of breathing is the most natural and basic of the breaths. It
can be practiced in a sitting or standing position as well as in a prone
position.

After mastering the *tanden* natural breath, you may proceed to the
next two breathing techniques.

(2)   Concentrated Breathing (Kumbhaka)
This breathing exercise may be done while either standing or sitting.
With the eyes open, concentrate your awarreness on a point in front of

you. Keep your eyes fixed on this point. Inhale, and then quickly exhale 10 percent. Hold the remaining 90 percent of the air in the abdomen and keep a good straight posture. When you no longer can hold the breath, release it. Continue this cycle of natural inhalation and holding of exhalation. This breathing exercise strengthens the body.

In the beginning, the tendency is to tighten the solar plexus. Please try to avoid tensing the body, especially in this region.

(3) *Palms Together Breathing* (Gasshō)

All religions practice palms together breathing. It unites the body and mind and prepares the person to listen to the voice from within. To perform *gasshō*, place the palms together in prayer position. The palms are held at a level higher than the heart. The elbows are raised in a straight line and point outward. The tip of the middle finger is level with the eyes. The eyes are half-closed, and concentration is on the tips of the fingers. Imagine that, when you inhale, the breath comes through the

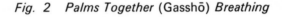

Fig. 2   Palms Together (Gasshō) *Breathing*

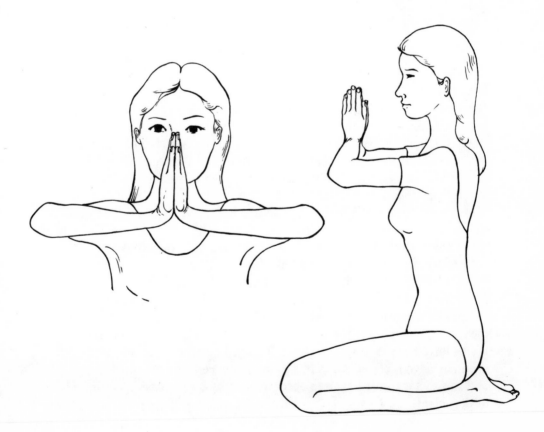

palms. Likewise, imagine that the exhalation goes out and upward through the base of the palms to the fingertips. Repeat this breathing cycle in a relaxed and natural way. After you master this breathing, you may perform the concentrated breathing technique in this position. With the palms together, practice holding the breath.

Gasshō breathing harmonizes imbalances between the sympathetic and parasympathetic nervous systems; thus this way of breathing calms the nervous system and promotes tranquility. If you continue *gasshō* breathing for more than thirty minutes, the hands will become very sensitive. You will feel much energy vibrating in the palm. This energy can be applied in a palm healing treatment.

When a person is in a healthy condition, his breathing is long and deep. Such a person will have a long life. When breathing is deep and clear, direction in life is purposeful and clear.

With practice and repeated training, physical habits are formed. In emergency situations these habits demonstrate their true value. If we train our breath to be long and deep, then we can remain calm in even the most stressful of situations.

Diet

The key to health and harmony can be found in our daily foods. A healthy person can eat almost anything he wants without any ill-effect. His choice of food, manner of preparation, volume and time of eating, however, must reflect an understanding of nature. He should know where his food comes from and for what purpose. He should study until he understands the power that is within food and the true reasons for eating. If he eats only to satisfy his desires, then imbalances will occur and he may lose his direction in life.

Our daily food is the foundation of our blood. Without a good foundation, even the mightiest of structures will crumble. Good blood quality is the cornerstone on which we build our health and our thinking.

Throughout history, mankind has always had the idea of a principle food. In the Far East, rice has been considered essential to man's well-being. In Central and South America, corn has been revered as the giver of life and nourishment. In North America and Europe, wheat has been the staple of every meal. For most people in the world, then, cereal grains have been the principle food. Today, however, meat and dairy products have replaced the cereal grain as the central part of the meal, and this dietary shift has been accompanied by an increasing occurrence of degenerative diseases.

To regain health and direction in our lives, then, we should eat a diet based on more time-honored staples. The macrobiotic diet reflects such a traditional approach, one that is based on a wide view of what is man and what is life. In general, it is suggested that we eat vegetable foods, choosing from whole cereal grains, vegetables (from both land and sea), beans, fruits and fermented foods such as *miso* and *tamari* soy sauce.

Our diet should reflect the natural order of things. It should be in harmony with the season, climate and our particular location on the earth. It should consider our activity, sex, age and dream. Our diet should change, as we change, to suit our needs and aid our development as whole persons.

After a period of eating well, the body begins to regain a state of natural understanding of its needs. This understanding is known as intuition. In the case of someone who has consumed great quantities of animal foods, sugar, drugs or chemicals, it will take a little while before his natural intuition returns.

The following guidelines will aid in the recovery of intuition:

1. Eat When Hungry, Drink When Thirsty. If we eat or drink too much or when the body has no need for food or drink, then we are not responding to our inner voice. Instead, we are indulging our sensorial appetite. Overindulgence in anything is harmful to one's well-being.

2. Choose and Eat Only Natural Whole Foods. Use whole unrefined foods as much as possible. Use whole grains, such as whole wheat, brown rice, millet, oats, corn, buckwheat, barley and rye. Choose vegetables that are fresh and chemical-free. Avoid processed, canned and frozen foods. Vegetables from the sea are rich in minerals and are very healthful.

3. Chew Well. Good food tastes better the more that one chews. Brown rice, for example, becomes sweeter when chewed well, whereas meat quickly loses its flavor. In this way, chewing also helps one to distinguish between good and bad food.

When one is sick, chewing well is essential. Digestion of complex carbohydrates begins in the mouth, so the more one chews, the better one's food is converted into nutrients usable by the body. To develop spirituality and sensitivity, it is also necessary to chew well. Mental clarity and judgment improves with mastication. In addition, complete chewing leads to satisfaction after a meal, and minimizes the desire to overeat.

4. *Eat Only to 80-percent Capacity:* Never eat until you are full. Overeating causes excess, which, if it is not discharged, will cause imbalance as more is taken in than is given off. Overeating brings the blood to the lower digestive regions of the body. It therefore takes blood away from the brain. As a consequence, clarity of thought is sacrificed through overindulgence. In order to respond accurately to the challenges of life, the mind must be alert. A person with a healthy appetite who eats only to 80-percent capacity can become very successful—his health will be secure and his direction will be clear.

5. *Enjoy Your Meals.* All food should be eaten with a spirit of gratitude and enjoyment.

6. *Do Not Eat When Upset.* If you are very tired, do not eat. If you are having emotional difficulties, do not eat. At these times the body is not prepared to receive food or to digest it properly and completely. At such times there is an excess of acid in the stomach, which will seriously affect one's digestive ability. In these circumstances, it is best to do something else before eating. Exercise or take a walk. Wait until you are calm.

7. *Your Kitchen Is Your Pharmacy.* Our daily food is our medicine. Thus the proper selection and preparation of daily meals is essential to the maintenance of health. Most illness, then, can be avoided with proper nutrition. If we eat well, we have no need for doctors.

Shin Do Fuji—"Body, Earth, Not Two"

The human body and the earth on which we live are not separate entities. If we think that we are separate from this earth, then already our attitude is incorrect.

In order to increase physical sensitivity and spiritual development, we must eat vegetable foods. We should avoid animal food, refined sugar (white or brown), honey and excessive amounts of fruits and fruit juices. Such foods interfere with our ability to feel and diagnose other people's conditions.

Thus, if we eat well, our understanding that we form an integrated unity with the earth will quickly develop. With this understanding our sensitivity will increase dramatically.

Exercise

The fundamental purpose of all exercise should be to develop one's native intuitive powers. Proper execution of the motions of an exercise is a way of harmonizing with the greater motions of the cosmos. If one moves smoothly, effortlessly and naturally, then one's movement can be said to be instinctive and balanced.

From birth until death, the life force is constantly in motion. According to Stieglitz (see Fig. 3), this movement manifests itself in four different ways: 1. intellectual ability; 2. sexual ability; 3. motor ability and 4. metabolic protective mechanism or unconscious survival ability.

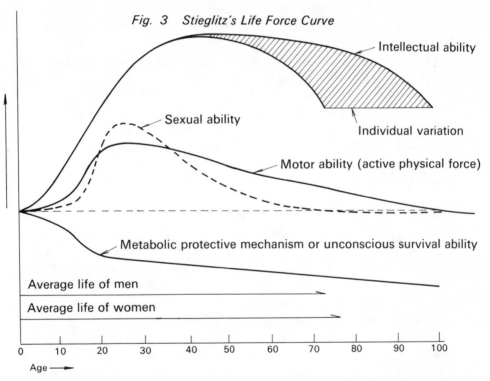

Fig. 3   Stieglitz's Life Force Curve

Intellectual ability increases with age and with study. Sexual ability increases gradually until about the age of twenty-two to twenty-five, and thereafter it declines. Motor ability develops gradually and evenly during one's lifetime, but begins to decrease after the age of thirty. In direct contrast to these three types of life-force changes, which increase to a peak in the course of one's life, the unconscious survival ability decreases steadily from the time of birth. The natural reflex action that we possess as children, for example, decreases as we get older. The body's resistance to disease decreases as well.

Exercise is important for maintaining all four abilities, especially the motor ability or active physical force. To perform an exercise well, three stages of motion must be well coordinated: its initiation, its maintenance and its control.

The point of doing exercises is not only to develop the muscles. Of course flexible muscles with good tone are of great value, but large muscles are not necessarily as asset. In order to successfully develop both mind and body in a balanced way, we must above all develop the three stages of motion.

The bones and muscles are responsible for the initiation of movement. Then, in order to sustain a movement we must have a strong breath. Lung capacity and circulation ability increase naturally with use. To develop coordination, though, one must exercise.

To develop our coordination we must challenge ourselves with our exercises. Our balance, for example, is controlled by our inner ear and brain. The simple act of standing is one exercise in balance. However, since it is such an everyday occurrence, it is no longer the challenge that it was when, as a child, we were learning to walk and stand upright. So in order to continue to develop our equilibrium, we must create new opportunities for balance; for example, by walking backward or with our eyes closed. The point is, if you already do something well, it will not develop you further to continue with easy exercises. You must choose difficult ones, for it is in meeting challenges that you develop.

According to Stieglitz's curve, the unconscious survival ability decreases after birth. To counteract this, we must train the autonomic nervous system to function in a balanced way. Throughout this book I stress the importance of proper breathing, proper food and proper attitude as well as exercises in daily living which will stimulate and challenge the brain and nervous system. If these tasks are performed well, one's intuition develops quickly and the automatic survival ability increases.

Man's flexibility is unmatched by any other animal and the coordination of his movements is truly remarkable. Twelve types of action are involved in the performance of his movement. Different exercises, of course, stress different actions. Such actions include: 1. bending forward and backward; 2. bending side to side; 3. twisting side to side; 4. moving up and down; 5. tensing and relaxing; 6. contracting and expanding (as in stretching). Each category of action contains two complementary movements. Thus all exercises can be said to be a combination of these six basic categories.

It is a common misconception that special equipment and a lot of space is needed to practice exercise and movement; on the contrary, very little is needed. To make muscles flexible and strong, they must be used. A gymnasium or baseball field is not a biological requirement for exer-

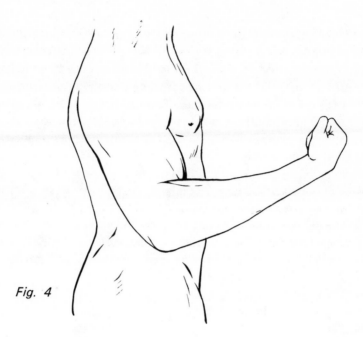

Fig. 4

cise. What is needed, however, is the desire to accomplish self-development.

If you want to develop any part of your body, put your concentration there. The voluntary muscles can be developed with a small amount of daily practice. For example, bring your attention to your arm. Inhale deeply into the *hara*. Make a strong contraction in the arm, and hold it for six to ten seconds. Exhale and relax. Repeat this exercise several times. (See Fig. 4.)

Imagine that you are carrying a large stone. With concentration on the action and with controlled breath, the muscles will respond as if you were actually lifting a heavy weight. Even if you are bedridden, you can practice this technique. In this way you can recover more quickly from your illness.

Skin Training Exercises

The skin is so directly related to the internal organs that it can be considered as a second heart or a second lung. The body's ability to cleanse itself of wastes is accomplished by the digestive and respiratory systems and by the skin.

a. Stimulate the skin daily with a brisk rub down with a stiff towel or brush. This will invigorate the skin, increasing its ability to breathe. It also increases the circulation.

b.   Take an air bath once or twice a day for about thirty minutes. Sit on a chair or on the floor. Open the window so that there is plenty of fresh air in the room. Keep the window open, even in winter time. Take off all your clothing and sit completely in the nude. In the beginning sit for ten seconds without any clothes. If you are cold, move your arms around and breathe deeply and quickly. After ten seconds, cover yourself with a blanket. When covered, just sit and make yourself warm for sixty seconds.

Begin again. This time increase nude time to twenty seconds. Cover up with the blanket for sixty seconds. Repeat this process, increasing the nude time by ten seconds each time. At sixty seconds of nude time, increase the blanket time to ninety seconds. When you reach the nude time of ninety seconds, you increase the blanket time to 120 seconds. Each day you can increase the time spent as you become stronger.

Fig. 5   How to Practice Air Bath

After six days basic training, practice twenty-seven minutes and twenty seconds. Accuracy is important.

	Cloth		Basic Training					
	Off	On						
	Second	Minute	First	Second	Third	Fourth	Fifth	Sixth
1	20 →	1						
2	30 →	1						
3	40 →	1						
4	50 →	1						
5	60 →	$1\frac{1}{2}$						
6	70 →	$1\frac{1}{2}$						
7	80 →	$1\frac{1}{2}$						
8	90 →	2						
9	100 →	2						
10	110 →	2						
11	120 →	On						

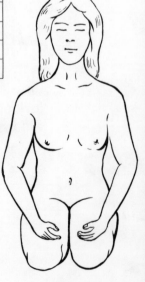

The best time to take an air bath is before sunrise and after sunset. If you are weak, you can do it during the daytime, but you should aim to do it during the dark time. Do not do this exercise thirty to forty minutes before or after meals. Continue taking air baths for thirty days, then rest for two to three days. Then continue for three months. If you have liver problems, continue repeatedly for one year. Cancer patients may perform this exercise frequently.

This skin training exercise is very effective and, in some instances, you may experience strong reactions. For example, some people get pimples, irritation, itchiness, skin color changes, etc. If these occur, you should not worry, for this is a normal reaction of the body as it adjusts. Sometimes air baths bring on dizziness, fever or coughing. Please continue, nevertheless, for these symptoms will disappear.

c. Substitute cold water in the air bath exercise. Enter cold water for ten seconds, then come out for one minute. Repeat with twenty seconds spent in the cold water, and so on.

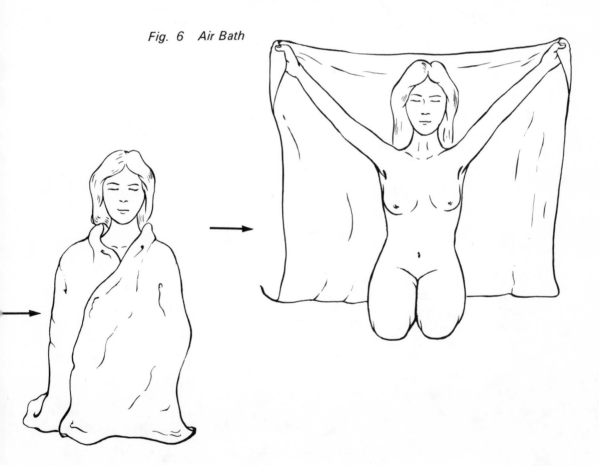

Fig. 6   Air Bath

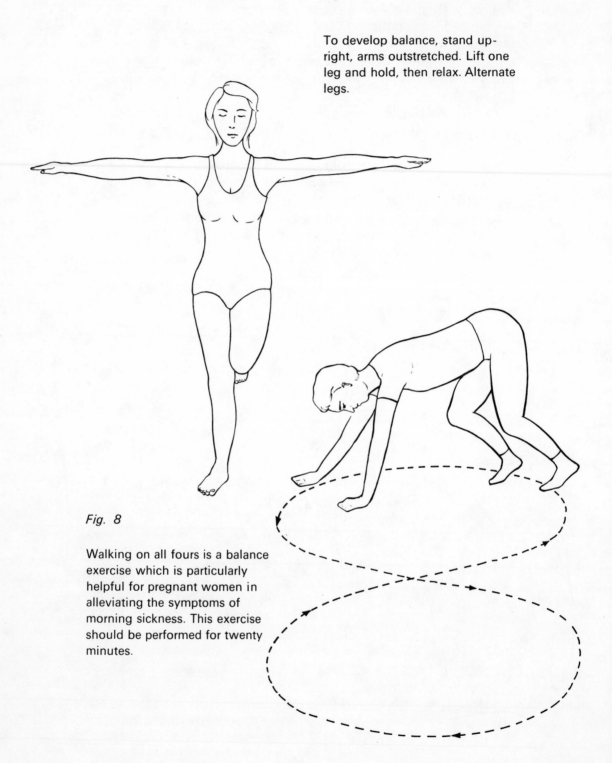

Fig. 7

To develop balance, stand upright, arms outstretched. Lift one
leg and hold, then relax. Alternate
legs.

Fig. 8

Walking on all fours is a balance
exercise which is particularly
helpful for pregnant women in
alleviating the symptoms of
morning sickness. This exercise
should be performed for twenty
minutes.

Balance Exercises

The best way to develop your balance is to use the parts of the body that you do not normally use. If your daily life demands that you sit all day, for example, then you must do balancing exercises that require the use of your legs. If you are accustomed to brushing your teeth with your right hand, begin using your left hand. Such exercises as the headstand, walking backward, standing on one leg, riding a skate board or a unicycle, or walking on all fours are useful in developing your balance.

Fig. 9

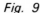

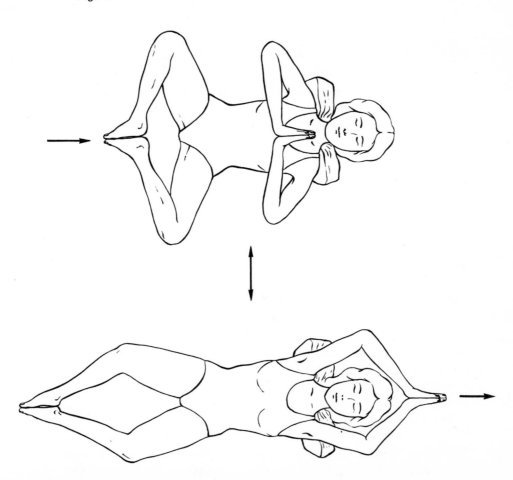

This exercise develops the balance and increases one's awareness of central coordination in the body. Lie on your back with your eyes closed. Bring your palms together and the soles of your feet together, stretch, inhale, exhale, then return both arms and legs toward the center. Repeat ten times.

Fig. 10

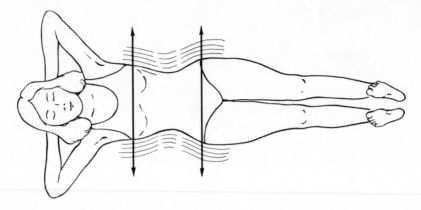

Roll the midbody back and forth to loosen the spine and help keep it flexible.

Cardiovascular Exercises

Exercises that have a beneficial effect on the heart and the blood vessels such as brisk walking, jogging, running, jumping rope, swimming and cycling are recommended. All exercises should be accompanied by controlled breathing.

Flexibility Exercises

All flexibility exercises help to correct the spine and to keep the body supple. Stretching and loosening exercises such as *tai-chi*, yoga, and *makkō-hō* are very valuable forms of flexibility training. Dancing is also recommended, although any stretching exercise is helpful.

Hara and Tanden Strengthening Exercises

If you train the *hara*, you will strengthen the whole body. That is why the martial arts focus on this vital area. All body movement, tension and relaxation originate from this region. If the lower abdomen is weak, you cannot move quickly. If the hip cannot relax, the whole body cannot relax.

The strength or weakness of the *tanden*, the central point in the *hara* region, is the mirror of the body's health. Coordination of the hips, abdominal muscles, and anus makes the *tanden* strong. The hip vertebrae must be straight, and, as they are movable, they should have a good ability to contract or expand. The abdominal muscles must also have strength and flexibility. The anus must have the power to contract strongly.

Fig. 11

To relax the hips and strengthen
the whole body, rotate the hip
area in a circular motion, first to
the left several times and then to
the right. Stretch the hips forward
and backward while bracing
against a wall.

Fig. 12

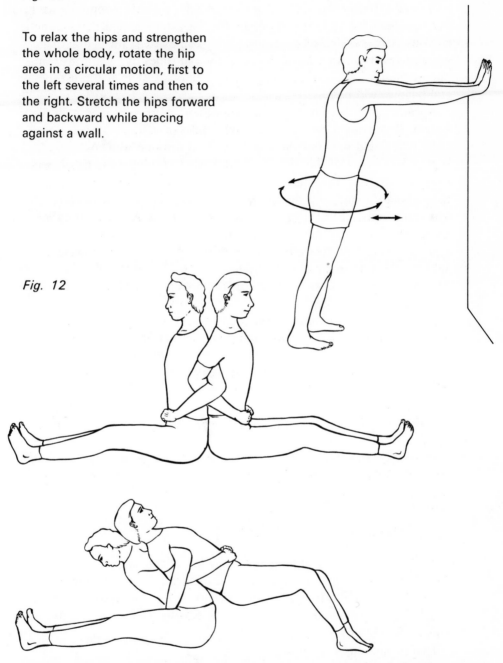

Exercise involving more than one person makes for good communication.
This back-to-back flexibility exercise stretches and loosens the spine, the
hips, and the *hara*, including the *tanden*.

The parasympathetic and sympathetic nervous systems work in a co-ordinated manner. When they function evenly, we have good balance in our bodies. If the body is not in balance, for example, if the sympathetic nervous system is overactive, no harmony can exist. If the sympathetic nervous system is used all of the time, then in times of need, for example, when attacked, the parasympathetic nervous system will not function and balance will be lost.

Normally it is thought that you cannot control the autonomic nervous system. If you could control it through an act of will, then when stress came you would remain calm and be able to respond well. Actually, it is possible to control this system. About one inch above the navel, and slightly to the left, the coeliac ganglion is located. This ganglion extends throughout the body via the splanchnic nerves. These nerves control the abdominal muscles as they spread throughout the *hara*, including the *tanden*. Therefore, by moving the abdomen through deep breathing and exercise you can stimulate the nerves of the parasympathetic nervous system. The autonomic nervous system also relates to the internal organs. Maintaining power in the *tanden* aids the organs in functioning well and helps maintain your health.

In our lives we need daily struggle. If we eat to capacity at every meal, if we live in air-conditioning in the summer and in well-heated homes during the winter, our nervous systems will not have the opportunity to develop and we will become weak and unhappy. If we are always warm and well-fed, if we are never challenged with difficulties, our lives will lack satisfaction and our health will quickly decline. We will become lazy and sick. We will not be in touch with the beauty that life brings.

If, on the other hand, we are interested in living an adventurous life, a life that abounds with energy and excitement, we had better develop our nervous systems.

Spontaneous Movement Technique

The effort to become healthy is not an action of the conscious mind. It is controlled by the autonomic nervous system. Therefore, the first prerequisite to health is to train the autonomic nervous system to respond automatically and sensitively, to the demands within the body. This is the aim of spontaneous movement.

Two preliminary exercises are:

a. While keeping the spine straight press the pit of the stomach with both hands and exhale. While exhaling, bend the upper body forward in an effort to exhale all the stagnant air remaining in the body. Repeat

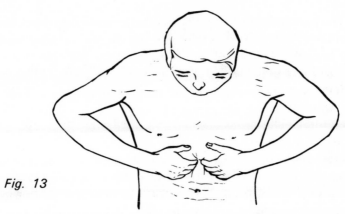

Fig. 13

twice. If the pit of the stomach becomes soft and if you yawn, let the yawn occur spontaneously. At this time you should breathe naturally (Fig. 13).

    b.   Regain a relaxed, straight back posture. This time stretch the upper body to the side as if you are looking at your own backbone. Twist to the left, release tension suddenly and return to the center. Relax the upper body, twist it to the right, release tension and suddenly return to normal. Go from side to side six times.

    These exercises are preparation for the practice of spontaneous movement. While exhaling slowly, open the palms, raise the arms and bend the body backward (Fig. 14). This stimulates the medula oblongata to

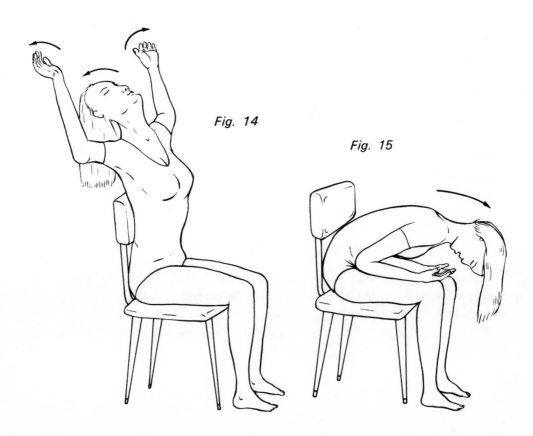

Fig. 14

Fig. 15

the small brain. Clench the molars and visualize strength pouring steadily into first the neck and then the backbone. Release this strength suddenly at its peak (Fig. 15). Repeat three times. (In natural life, inhalation involves an intake of strength, and exhalation a release of strength. In this training exercise, however, we do it in reverse order to stimulate the autonomic nervous system along the backbone all the way to the small brain.)

Still seated, place your hands, palms up, on the knees and close your eyes. Drop your head and imagine yourself breathing into your backbone, or think of yourself as actually breathing with your backbone. You may feel your body start moving, just let it move. Try to breathe into the part of your body that is moving, so the movement will become bigger. If the neck moves, for example, you breathe into the neck. Do not deliberately move any part of your body. This involuntary movement may become so big that it may not cease even if you try to stop it. It may last for a long time. Just allow the movement to go its own way without trying to stop it, for it will come to a stop eventually by itself.

When the movement comes to a stop, remain quietly with your eyes closed for one or two minutes. The empty or quiet feeling in your mind which comes just after spontaneous movement is entirely different from absent-mindedness at other times.

To stop the movement after it has started, breathe into your stomach and hold your breath. Gradually, the movement will come to a standstill. Then return to ordinary breathing. When you have opened your eyes, breathe into your stomach quietly once again. Controlling your breath, exhale slowly. That is all you have to do.

Timing (*Ma Ai*)

The practices of proper breathing, diet and exercise are all essential for the development of the whole person. *Ki Ketsu Dō* is the art of developing and utilizing ki, the life force of the universe, and ketsu, a superior blood quality. Breathing, diet and exercise develop ki and ketsu.

A fourth practice is needed in order to function as a free human being. This is timing, the knowledge of when to respond and when not to respond to the external environment. The Japanese concept of *Ma Ai* concerns itself with the coordination of this distance between one's self and one's surroundings. *Ma* means distance and *Ai* means union. In the case of shiatsu treatment, one must attune one's self to the recipient's condition in order to really make contact. For me to talk to you, for example, I must speak at a time when I know that you will be listening. In other words, I must coordinate my speaking with your ability to listen.

The art of *Ma Ai*, then, must be developed to ensure successful treatment. When *Ma Ai* is good, a proper distance is maintained between giver and receiver, a distance which permits effective treatment but at the same time ensures a feeling of oneness. Thus when one's timing is good, one will not be bound by immediate circumstances; hence one's judgment will be accurate.

You must be healthier than or superior to those whom you treat. The development of *Ma Ai* makes you a little bit superior to those around you. If you are not stronger than they are, they will not feel satisfied by your treatment. When you learn to coordinate the distance between yourself and another and are superior to him, then you can stimulate that other person to heal himself. It is to accomplish this goal that we train.

Meditation

If we place our concentration on our inner voice, we respond naturally to the world around us and we feel ourselves to be an integral part of a greater whole. We must always maintain such feelings of belonging. This is the goal and practice of meditation.

Meditation should occur in one's daily life. In other words it is not necessary to sit and think in order to meditate. Instead, one should concentrate on developing one's feeling for what life is by investigating one's relationship with the universe. When one understands that we were made by nature and are living in nature, then one can naturally understand the reason why we are here. From this sort of meditation one comes to understand that we are all friends and that we are all here to help each other.

Nevertheless, we must recognize that man is fundamentally an independent creature, for he is born alone and dies alone. Thus his primary responsibility must be placed in himself. This of course does not mean that he should ignore those around him, for if he recognizes that they too make up the whole, then naturally he will direct his energy toward helping his fellow man. To do this most effectively, however, he should be centered during every minute of his daily life, for it is only from a centered position that he can effectively choose and operate in the world. To find his center, he must meditate.

In itself, of course, the act of meditation has no intrinsic value. The technique of sitting with a straight posture alone does not ensure one's development. Nevertheless, correct posture is very important, especially when one is self-reflecting. Both the *seiza* posture and full lotus posture are very good for this purpose. One should sit completely relaxed, as though planted between heaven and earth. At this time, the body and mind should be completely relaxed and the spine should be held straight. If the body slumps forward or backward, the natural flow of energy is impeded and the nervous system is stressed. As a consequence, the thoughts which result from such a posture will be a reflection of that stress itself, rather than of one's true nature.

Every minute is meditation. To develop your meditative powers, be attentive to the world around you. In this way, little by little you will come to understand your true relationship to the universe. This is the dynamic way of meditation.

Hara

Everything on this earth has a balancing point and in man this finds its place in the *hara*, the place from which his vitality originates. If an object's balancing point is close to the ground, it is stable and cannot easily be knocked over. Similarly, when a man's consciousness is centered in the *hara*, he feels very stable. At the same time he feels abounding energy.

We must practice allowing our center of gravity to come down to this one point. Most modern people concentrate their energies on thinking, and thus they always keep their energy up in their heads. They tend to overemphasize the importance of thought while neglecting the body, the biological foundation of their thinking. This manifests itself most dramatically in their tendency to strengthen the upper portions of their bodies such as the arms and the shoulders, while neglecting the hips and the lower regions. However, the hip is the foundation of the body and unless it is strong, the body will weaken. A weak foundation will not stand long; the simplest stress will bring it crashing down.

All actions should naturally be performed from the *hara*. In Japan, for example, *Noh* drama, calligraphy, *sumi-e* brush painting, flower arranging, tea ceremony and the martial arts are practiced with the attention focused there. Similarly, shiatsu becomes most effective when one's movements originate from the *hara*.

Hara is the physical center of the body and so it must be strengthened. It is here that digestion occurs and it is here that food is broken down and converted into energy. In terms of the yogic *chakra* system, the *hara* is the region where the body's physical charge is centered. When the charge is strong, so is the rest of the body. Interestingly enough, it is in this region that the developing embryo grows. Here the fetus receives the strong physical charge vital in its early growth.

Ki

Although the Japanese word *ki* may be unfamiliar to many Westerners, the concept itself is not. Ki is a term used to name the life force of the universe. Everything that exists was created by ki. Ki has no beginning and no end; it is vibration. It cannot be understood with the mind by analysis. Ki is equal to energy, spirit, and mind.

The ancient healing systems of China, India, Greece, and Japan recognized the importance of both the material and the spiritual in the care of disease. But more recently, especially in the West, there has been a decline in this outlook which combines body and mind. This century's investigation has emphasized the importance of matter. Today many people feel that to own material things is of the utmost importance. In some cases, they feel that an understanding of life will come through materialism. This attitude is reaching its peak. At the same time we are beginning to return to vitalism or to the understanding that ki is also important.

The concept of a life force first appeared nearly 5,000 years ago. It was written about in China in the *Nei Ching* 4,500 years ago. Yoga texts from India refer to a vital life force that was known about 4,000 years ago. Over 2,500 years ago Socrates said you should cure with a look at the entire condition: "Just as you ought not to attempt to cure eyes without head or head without body, so you should not treat body without soul."

Ki fills all things that exist. When someone is very active and radiates a healthy look, you can be sure that you are witnessing ki. Like everything in the universe, ki changes constantly according to the order of the universe. As long as you are alive, you must continue to receive ki. When ki flows smoothly in the body all the organs and functions go well. If ki flows sluggishly, you feel weak and tired and finally become ill. In shiatsu we stimulate the body so it will receive and utilize ki. In this way we can revitalize and so effect a cure.

The term ki is used in many ways in the Japanese language. "I like you" is said *Ki ni iru,* or "It suits my ki." Sickness is *byō ki* meaning "ki got sick." When two friends are in harmony, it is said *Ki ga au* or "ki meets together."

2. The Unique Attitude of Barefoot Shiatsu

Massage is one of the oldest and most instinctual of healing practices and has been used since mankind's earliest beginnings. Over 4,500 years ago, massage was recorded in the *Nei Ching* or *The Yellow Emperor's Classic of Internal Medicine*. This treatise on medicine is still used today in China, the land of its origin. The art of massage has evolved into a variety of highly specialized and diversified methods, one of which is shiatsu.

In the ancient texts of oriental medicine it is written that mankind and nature are one; that is, both are part of the great universe.

Separation from nature brings a feeling of alienation and the beginning of physical, emotional and psychological disease. Nature is in a state of continuous change. We can very easily understand this as we observe the daily change from day to night, or the continuous flow of one season into the next, winter into spring, summer into fall. When we feel separate from this great order of universal change, we are experiencing disease.

The unique attitude of shiatsu is to remind man of the source of his disharmony. It is relatively easy to eliminate symptoms of illness, such as aches and pains. However, this is not the true purpose of shiatsu. Shiatsu treatment is aimed at making man whole. That is, the purpose of shiatsu is to re-establish the harmony between man and the universe.

Shiatsu never seeks to cure the patient. The patient must heal himself. The practitioner is only the stimulus to aid the patient in assuming a proper direction. The practitioner serves as a mirror for the patient, allowing the patient the opportunity to self-reflect on the true cause of his condition.

In order to achieve a lasting cure—that is, to create a life that is full and vigorous, without mental, emotional or physical imbalances—harmony with nature is essential. Shiatsu treatment gives the patient a clear direction to follow.

Sickness is neither good nor bad. It is a warning from the universe that informs us of disharmony and imbalance in our ego-centered life-style. This is a naturally protective mechanism.

The intelligent person listens to this information and reflects deeply on the causes of the spiritual, emotional, psychological, and physical problems that exist. We cannot separate the psychological from the physical, just as we cannot separate the mind from the body.

Body and Mind

When you think of body and mind, do you not first think of two separate entities? It is easy to think of the body. The body has substance and is finite. With the mind it is not always so easy. The mind has no color, shape or limits; still we all know that it exists. It is easy to perceive an unhealthy body, but how can we see an unhealthy mind? Although at first we think that body and mind are separate, at the same time we feel that, actually, this may not be so. The intangible aspects of a person's being, such as intelligence, emotion, memory, etc. have a direct influence on the function of the mind. Mind and body reflect the condition of each other. It is the aim of shiatsu to encourage the patient to readjust his life-style, thus bringing about a unification of body and mind. Both body and mind originate from the ki of the universe and are ultimately one. As practitioners of shiatsu, we must be attentive to the condition of our bodies and minds. When the two are unified, a clear channel is created for the healing force to move through us.

Natural Healing Uses Natural Power

Our technique tries to assist the body in healing itself. The patient is the actual healer. Generally, the shiatsu practitioner applies approximately 80–90 percent effort to the patient. Never does he give a 100 percent effort. If we did apply 100 percent the body would not be given the chance to build and develop its own natural healing power. By using only 80–90 percent we allow external ki to enter the receiver. This is enough to assist the body in its present condition.

Harmony

"Nature abhors a vacuum." For example warm air rises, therefore leaving space for cooler air to fill. During summer, cool sea breezes come to the warmer land masses. Water always flows downward until it meets the ocean. What are these natural processes? Are they not examples of nature seeking harmony? If there is a condition of imbalance, for example one area is warmer than another, then nature seeks to establish equilibrium or to make a balance with this inequality. This movement goes on constantly. The dictionary tells us that harmony is "completeness and perfection resulting from diversity in unity; orderliness." Everything in nature seeks harmony; so too our bodies seek balance and harmony. All sickness is an attempt to reestablish balance.

Oriental and Western Approaches to Healing

Acupuncture is currently very popular. This system is based on the theory that energy flows through set pathways in the body. If there is a blockage in this flow of energy, it is reflected as an imbalance in the body. This blockage manifests itself externally as pain or soreness which reflects internal malfunctioning of the associated organs. Acupuncturists and acupuncture textbooks see the study of meridians as essential to effective treatment. Indeed, without knowledge of the exact locations of a pressure point along a meridian, the acupuncturist would not know where to insert the needle, and the treatment would be ineffective or even harmful.

In addition to an intensive study of acupuncture points and meridians, the acupuncturist must undertake a study of the pulses. One can diagnose the body's condition from the taking of twelve pulses, six in each wrist. In order to be effective and to truly understand these techniques, years of study and practice are required.

Shiatsu is also based on the concepts of traditional oriental medicine, but its approach is much simpler than that of acupuncture; shiatsu uses a direct, instinctive approach. It is not necessary to learn pulse diagnosis or to study the meridian system extensively. Reality is very simple and direct; similarly, effective shiatsu treatment is simple and direct.

To become an effective shiatsu practitioner, one must satisfy the following:

1. One must develop sensitivity.
2. One must develop one's self psychologically, emotionally and physically.
3. One must have knowledge and experience.

A curious, healthy person will automatically fulfill these requirements. This is the natural way. It is the common sense approach. By completely developing yourself, your sensitivity naturally increases.

Along with instinctual sensitivity comes the curiosity for information. This curiosity is satisfied with study and experience. You should be aware of the oriental approach to medicine which sees life as a whole. All sickness occurs because there is an imbalance. The most direct apillness. proach to health considers the way of life as both the cause and the cure of illness. Also, our knowledge must include the latest scientific information. There is nothing outside of the whole. Western scientific information does not conflict with the oriental approach. Information is information no matter what the source. However, the usual western approach is to divide into fragments, that is, to observe the parts without considering the whole. For this reason, western medicine treats the symptoms rather than the cause.

Shiatsu combines the scientific approach with the oriental-traditional holistic approach. Today many practitioners of oriental medicine use western techniques, such as naming illnesses. In shiatsu, naming, though not essential to the cure, is useful at times. It is my hope that oriental practitioners will study and understand the western approach, and that allopathic, western-style doctors will learn the ancient oriental approach.

Health

Health is more than merely being without sickness. It is a dynamic state in which the mental, physical and spiritual lives harmonize. The key to health is prevention (*yōjyō* in Japanese). The intelligent person always

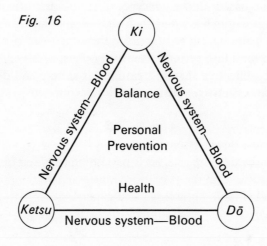

Fig. 16

prevents unnecessary hardships from arising. Oriental medicine is based on this concept of prevention. In Japan there is a saying: "*Ki ketsu ei ei.*" This is the formula for good health. *Ki* is life force, *ketsu* is good quality blood, and *ei ei* is proper nourishment. Our daily food, being proper human nourishment, will make good quality blood. Ki flows in a body with good quality blood.

Past, Present and Future Health

Past actions have created the present health and what we do today will determine how we feel in the future. We must begin to understand ourselves from this fundamental viewpoint. Our general physical and mental tendencies originate in our daily habits. Our past and present dietary practice, physical exercise, mental activity and our general view of life have created our present state of health and condition our future health. If an harmonious state of health has been lost, it is the responsibility of the patient to regain it. The shiatsu practitioner is only the channel through which stimulus to change emerges. Direction comes from the practitioner; action comes from the patient.

Fatigue

A healthy person who uses his entire body in the course of daily activities will, from time to time, experience fatigue, the pleasurable feeling of having worked hard. At the end of the day, the whole body can relax and recuperate. Such fatigue is good. It is the slowing-down process from a job well done. It is a reward for good work. Actually, this is not fatigue but the second half of all activity: rest, the body's response to exertion.

Another real fatigue that is common today is mental, emotional and physical exhaustion or weariness before any physical work is done. Many people wake up in the morning after a night of disturbed sleep to find themselves more tired than when they went to bed. Daily tasks of cleaning the house or even family outings exhaust and weaken them. Why do people suffer from fatigue?

Improper Use of the Body

Using the body in an unbalanced way will strain it and deplete its vital life force. If you use one part of your body exclusively and neglect other parts—for example, always using the right hand and arm—the energy flow within the body will be unilateral. Also, after exertion it is necessary to allow the body time to recuperate. Without recuperation, the biological functions connected with cleansing the blood will be unable to do their job completely; and a state of fatigue will persist.

Relaxation Technique: Do you not think it is strange that we must learn to relax? Because our daily lives are filled with doing, it is important to spend some time in nonactivity. If during the day, you participate completely in your activities with an undivided body and mind, naturally rest and relaxation will occur. Few of us, however, allow ourselves the apparent luxury of living a complete life; that is, a life in which both body and mind do the same thing at the same time.

The easiest way to achieve relaxation is to be physically active. It is good to perform some activity each day, such as taking a long walk, gardening, jogging, swimming, etc. However, after the performance of such exercise it is important to relax completely. To achieve deep relaxation, lie on your back and begin to breathe into your *hara*. Allow air and the energy it brings to saturate the area. Next, contract the toe muscles, then exhale and relax. Move your awareness up the legs to the knees, contract them, and then exhale and relax. Relaxation always comes at exhalation. Move your awareness up the legs to the thighs, contracting and then relaxing. Continue to the buttocks, the abdomen, the chest, neck and shoulders. Then contract and relax the fingers, the wrists, the forearms, and the upper arms. Allow the relaxing energy from the breath to enter the head and face region. Contract the face muscles and relax them. Finally, tense the whole body and hold this position. Hold it a little longer, still longer, until at last you must let go and allow energy to fill and soothe the entire body. Remain in this relaxed state until you naturally feel it is time to return to your activities.

Improper Breathing

Without slow, deep breathing, the body will lack oxygen.

Improper Diet

The combination of good food and oxygen brings complete digestion, which in turn creates sufficient energy for the organism.

Emotional and Psychological Imbalance

Situations fraught with emotional and psychological stress drain the body of its energy supply and cause fatigue.

Lack of Adaptability

The inability to respond and adapt to life's changes can also cause fatigue; for example, if you travel to a foreign country, you must adjust to its customs and food. If you do not adapt willingly, sickness may force you. Similarly, if you use your body and mind completely in your daily life, you will experience little or no fatigue. If you do office work for example, then you should dance or do physical work to balance it. In other words you must know yourself and make variety in your daily routine.

Oriental Medicine's View of the Causes of Sickness

Why do we get sick? The oriental approach to illness is an holistic one. It divides the causes for illness into two: those influences which come from the inside and those influences which come from the outside.

Naishō Influences Which Come from Inside the Body

A. *The Five Emotional Causes of Sickness*
  (1) Excess of joy, pleasure or delight causes heart trouble.
  (2) Excess of anger damages the liver.
  (3) Excess melancholy or sadness damages the stomach, spleen, or pancreas.
  (4) Excess grief harms the lungs.
  (5) Fear and surprise harm the kidneys.
These emotional conditions cause fatigue and sickness. In addition, too much stimulation causes imbalance in the nervous system.

B. *The Five Tastes*
The proper amount of a particular taste is beneficial to its associated organ. Excess of the same flavor, however, damages the very organ that a smaller amount benefits. In other words, we must always take enough, but not too much. Such is the order of the universe.
  (1) The sour flavor is good for the liver, but too much sourness damages it as well as hurting the stomach, spleen, and pancreas. Sourness loosens the body.
  (2) The bitter flavor is good for the heart. An excess of this flavor, however, damages the heart and the lungs. Bitter flavor causes contraction. It acts as a laxative, aiding the discharge of excess.
  (3) The sweet flavor in small amounts is good for the stomach, spleen

and pancreas. In excess, though, the sweet flavor damages these organs as well as the kidneys, teeth and bones. Sweetness has a dispersing effect and, when taken in moderation, it has a relaxing effect.

(4)   A pungent flavor (hot and spicy) is good for the lungs. In excess it damages the lungs and liver. It has an upward, dispersing effect.

(5)   In proper amounts salt is good for the kidneys, but in excess it damages the kidneys and heart. The salt taste causes contraction.

Among the five tastes, salty and sweet are the easiest to overindulge. It is through the use of salt and sweeteners that many sicknesses and troubles come about. If someone who is already sick takes an excess of either sugar or salt, it will aggravate the symptoms.

Salt: A proper amount of salt suited to your personal condition, activity, and the time of year, acts as a source of energy, strengthening the kidney, heart and liver functions. It will improve circulation and aid the functioning of the hormone system. Too little or too much salt, however, lowers your vitality.

A person who eats, or has eaten in the past, large amounts of animal food does not require much salt, since meat and animal products contain a high amount of sodium. Heavy intake of animal food after childbirth causes a tightening inside the body, which impedes normal discharging. Animal food causes a quantity of mucus which, if retained, will cause post-delivery problems. In ancient Japan, for seven days after the delivery of child, the new mother was given only vegetable foods. If a *yin*-type person wants to become *yang* and eats plenty of salt in an attempt to accomplish this goal, his body will become increasingly stiff. The kidneys will contract and will not function well, and his mentality will become rigid.

A heavy intake of salt impedes healing in the following illnesses: acute nephritis, pleurisy, pneumonia, pulmonary troubles, conjunctivitis, inflammation of the middle ear, sinusitis, tonsilitis, dermatitis, skin eruptions, hepatitis, jaundice, appendicitis, cystitis, gonorrhea, stomatitis and acute feverish, contagious disease conditions. Too much salt is also harmful in the case of infectious diseases, such as measles, dysentery, typhoid fever, acute gastritis, influenza and whooping cough. If someone with a fever takes too much salt the fever will be held inside the body.

Sugar: Like too much salt, overconsumption of sugar leads to serious health problems. Today, many people are decreasing, or eliminating, consumption of refined, white sugar. This is commendable and urgently necessary. Most brown sugar is white sugar with 6–8 percent molasses

added for color. All so-called natural sugars—turbinado and raw sugar—
are almost identical to refined white sugar. In the United States, it is law
that all sugars must be processed. The sweet flavor also is found in fruits,
honey and maple syrup. All of the above sweeteners are very strong.

Small amounts of good quality sweetness, as found in cooked carrots,
squash, and cereal grains, will help the stomach, spleen, and pancreas.
Such sweetness is good for the muscles. It stimulates kidney function
and therefore makes one more energetic. It also aids lung function. It is
also good for ki ketsu circulation, the combined circulation of blood
and life force. Consumption of such naturally sweet foods also aids in
growth and in the proper functioning of the hormone system.

Complex carbohydrates are the best source of sugar. If you eat grains,
which are complex carbohydrates, you will not suffer from lack of sugar
as it is. This kind of sugar is broken down and utilized slowly by the
body; and as a consequence the pancreas is not overstimulated as is by
simpler sugars like honey. Energy is released steadily from complex
carbohydrates; there is no rush and then a letdown. Normally special
sugar supplements are unnecessary, unless you do very hard physical
work, in which case you may want a little added sugar in the form of
dried fruits or grain syrups such as "Yinnies," or barley malt. Mountain
climbers enjoy the boost these simpler sugars give.

Sugar has an expansive function. Too much of it loosens the whole
body, lowers all functioning, and causes processes of degeneration ending
in numbness. Excess sugar causes problems in the stomach, spleen and
pancreas. As a result the kidneys must overwork, skin color becomes
reddish or blackish, and blemishes tend to appear. An unreasonable
amount of sugar spoils the teeth and bones by robbing them of such
minerals as calcium for sugar metabolism. The lungs cannot function
well, and the metabolic rate drops. It is easier to catch cold or to get
tuberculosis. Excess sugar consumption is a pre-condition for all yin
diseases, including the following: acute gastritis, hyperacidity and gastric
ulcer. Chronic conditions include the dropping of the internal organs on
the uterus, frigidity in females, cervical cancer, beriberi, amnesia, tuberculosis, dental caries, decayed teeth, myopia, diabetes mellitus, polio,
leukemia, paralysis, rheumatism, muscular dystrophy and multiple
sclerosis.

Children are small and compact. It is natural for them to grow or
expand. So it is natural for children to like sweet things. But it is important to educate them to enjoy the proper, nourishing sweets that
satisfy and aid growth. Refined white sugar and similar sweeteners are
not good for children. If children eat too much of them they will grow
like; bean sprouts: very fast, but without physical strength. They will
have dental cavities and bone problems. Sugar increases the likelihood

of scrofula, or a predisposition to glandular tumors.

C. *Poisons: Food, Water, and* Oketsu *(Mucus)*

We have already discussed some food poisons—excess intake of sugar and salt. With overeating and drinking, undigested food remains in the intestines. This promotes fermentation that produces toxins that enter the blood, causing acidosis. Even overdoses of alkaline foods such as raw vegetables cause acidosis, which may be either acute or chronic.

Water poisoning is caused by excessive intake of such yin type food as fruits, raw vegetables, and liquid. In this case the blood becomes too alkaline. Excessive liquid or sugar consumption upsets the digestive and urinary systems.

In *oketsu*, a condition that occurs mainly in females instead of naturally discharging accumulated waste, the body retains the bad quality blood resulting from excessive amounts of mucus in the body. Such excess blocks and congests the flow of energy and body fluids. The entire body becomes very stagnant as mucus in the kidneys interferes with blood filtration. This mucus may harden to form cysts or stones. In such cases, ki does not flow well and many organs do not function well.

Female problems, like headache, low abdominal pain, palpitations of the heart, sleeplessness, fear, melancholy and nervous troubles, often result from *oketsu*. There are several causes of this mucus-retention condition. After childbirth, the mother should rest for three weeks. Without enough recuperation time, the body cannot completely cleanse itself. In addition, she should refrain from sexual intercourse for approximately three months. Sexual experience before this time may cause *oketsu*, which may also occur after an abortion.

The excess blood in a woman's body is normally discharged monthly with the menstrual cycle or after the delivery of a child. When this cleansing process does not occur, or when incomplete menstruation causes bleeding between periods (a condition more prevalent than cancer), waste remains in the body and finds its way into the blood. In this way, the woman is poisoned from the inside.

What impedes this normal protective function? Too much emotional stress together with excessive intake of animal food and sugar causes *oketsu* to remain in the body. The *oketsu* condition is a serious cause of fatigue that can lead to many other troubles.

D. *Go-Rō Shichi-Shō (Five Overexertions Cause Seven Spoiled Conditions)*

(1) Long-time working damages the liver.

(2) Long-time focusing of the eyes, like reading, damages the circu-

lation and the heart.

(3) Long-time sitting damages the muscles and causes spleen and pancreas trouble.

(4) Long-time standing damages the bones and produces kidney trouble.

(5) Long-time lying down damages ki flow and causes lung problems.

In addition to these five overexertions, we would like to add two more:

(1) Excessive eating and drinking damages the stomach.

(2) Too much sexual activity damages the kidney and overworks the heart.

Gaija Influences Which Come from Outside the Body

An excessive exposure to wind, cold, heat, humidity and dryness can cause illness. These natural conditions can be considered external stress.

Classical oriental medicine views both internal and external influences as the primary causes of illness. Illness develops in stages. The first stage is increasing fatigue and tiredness. If someone complains of fatigue, we know this symptom indicates that something is going wrong in the body.

To treat only the symptom is partial treatment. Fatigue and sickness are intimately related to life-style. Thus one must search for the cause rather than merely noticing and reacting to the symptom. In this way one treats the person in his entirety. This includes a consideration of the person's way of life.

Autonomic Nervous System

The nervous system, which controls all bodily actions and operations, is divided into two major systems: the central nervous system which consists of the brain and the spinal cord, and the autonomic nervous system which regulates the functioning of such internal organs as the stomach, intestines, heart, womb, glands, and so on.

The autonomic nervous system consists of the sympathetic nervous system and the parasympathetic nervous system. It is located in the spinal cord and the brain stem. One set of nerves causes activity in the smooth muscles of the body, the other set reverses this activity (see Fig. 17). All illness and imbalance affects the autonomic nervous system.

54

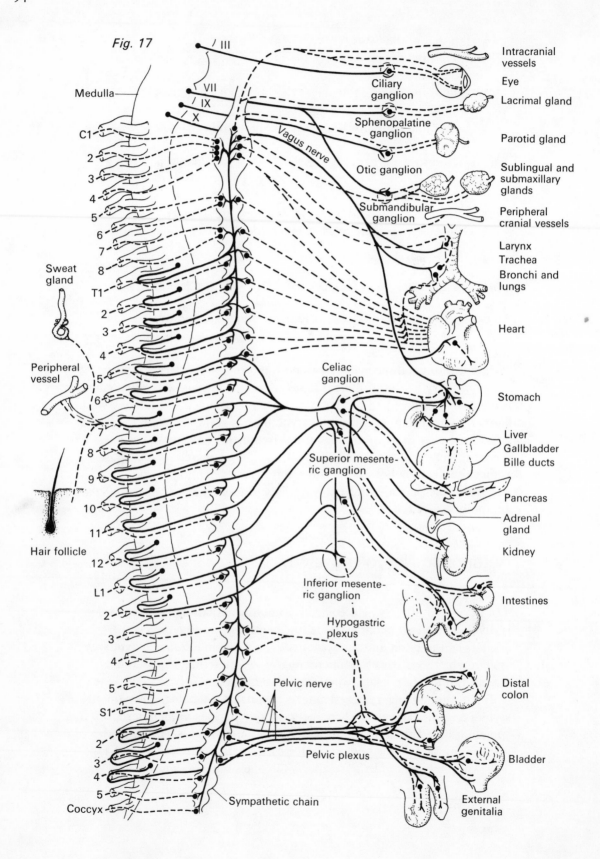

Fig. 17

Medulla

Sweat gland

Peripheral vessel

Hair follicle

C1
2
3
4
5
6
7
8
T1
2
3
4
5
6
7
8
9
10
11
12
L1
2
3
4
5
S1
2
3
4
5
Coccyx

III
VII
IX
X

Vagus nerve

Ciliary ganglion

Sphenopalatine ganglion

Otic ganglion

Submandibular ganglion

Celiac ganglion

Superior mesenteric ganglion

Inferior mesenteric ganglion

Hypogastric plexus

Pelvic nerve

Pelvic plexus

Sympathetic chain

Intracranial vessels

Eye

Lacrimal gland

Parotid gland

Sublingual and submaxillary glands

Peripheral cranial vessels

Larynx
Trachea
Bronchi and lungs

Heart

Stomach

Liver
Gallbladder
Bille ducts

Pancreas

Adrenal gland

Kidney

Intestines

Distal colon

Bladder

External genitalia

Autonomic Nervous System

	Sympathetic Nervous System (Yin)	Parasympathetic Nervous System (Yang)
Smooth muscle	activates	deactivates
Eye pupil	dilates	contracts
Salivary glands	produces less, thicker saliva	produces more, thinner saliva
Windpipe	opens	contracts
Liver	activates sugar digestion	deactivates sugar digestion
Heart	beats faster	beats slower
Skin	loosens	contracts (causing goose flesh)
Blood vessel	contracts	dilates
Blood pressure	increases	lowers
Spleen	activates	does not affect
Digestive system	deactivates	activates
Adrenal glands	produces more adrenalin	influence is slight
Penis	contracts blood vessels, so no erection	expands blood vessels, so more erection
Bladder	loosens	contracts
Sweat glands	thicker perspiration	thinner perspiration

Supreme health is based on an equilibrium between its two branches. This balance can be accomplished by barefoot shiatsu.

In the 1930's the Canadian Hans Selye theorized that an imbalance in the autonomic nervous system is the basic cause of all diseases. He felt that one would not suffer illness if the two branches of the autonomic nervous system were in harmony. Similarly, in the 1950's, a Frenchman named Dr. Reilly studied the mechanism of hormone secretion and found that they are made directly upon order from the interbrain. He thought that if one's interbrain was in good condition then one would not contract disease.

There is an interesting connection between the nervous system in the body and the meridian system of ancient oriental medicine. Fig. 17 shows this relationship very clearly. Along the spinal column there are many nerve branches that lead to various internal organs. Ancient oriental medicine recognized this direct relationship between the spine and the internal organs. The bladder meridian, which connects with all the internal organs, runs along the spine. By treating this meridian along the spine, the ancients reasoned, one could influence specific organ functions.

Fig. 18   Twelve Major Points on the Bladder Meridian

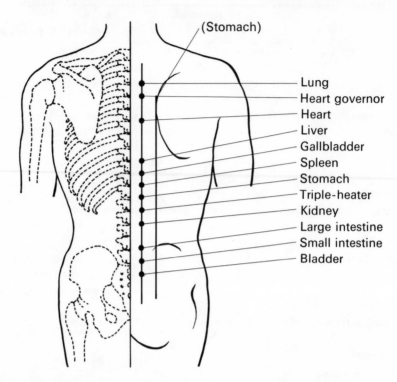

(Stomach)

Lung
Heart governor
Heart
Liver
Gallbladder
Spleen
Stomach
Triple-heater
Kidney
Large intestine
Small intestine
Bladder

The relationship between the body surface and the internal organs can be used very profitably in shiatsu therapy. Diagnosis and treatment are one and the same. Following the pathway down the center of the back, the therapist can discover points of sensitivity—locations of pain or dullness, heat or cold, protrusions or indentations. It is possible to feel whether the points are full (*jitsu*) or empty (*kyo*). Each point corresponds to the functioning of an internal organ. Once you have discovered them, you can correct the malfunctioning organ by stimulating the applicable external points. (See Fig. 18, which lists the twelve major points on the bladder meridian.)

Proper functioning of the autonomic nervous system and unrestricted flow of ki energy throughout the body will strengthen the body. Balance between the nervous system and the flow of life force in the body protects health.

Sometimes conditions arise in the body that necessitate consultation with a doctor. After the checkup, if there has been no apparent cause of the condition, such as an accident, operation or extremely adverse weather conditions, the doctor may not be able to make a diagnosis. In such cases the cause is probably a malfunctioning of the autonomic nervous system.

An imbalance in the working of the sympathetic and parasympathetic branches can cause the following symptoms or feelings:

1. Ringing in the ears
2. Worry about the heartbeat
3. Tight, constricted feeling in the upper chest area
4. Rapid heartbeat
5. Breathing difficulty
6. Feeling that one's breath is shorter than other people's
7. Shortness of breath even while resting
8. Cold hands even in summer
9. Coldness or purple coloration of the fingertips
10. Constant lack of appetite
11. Feeling of nausea
12. Constant worry about digestion
13. Weak digestion
14. Stomach pain when hungry or after eating
15. Chronic diarrhea or constipation
16. Stiff neck
17. Tiredness of the limbs
18. Hypersensitive skin
19. Frequent redness of the face
20. Excess perspiration, even in winter
21. Occasional skin rash
22. Continual headaches
23. Sudden chills or sensations of heat
24. Occasional loss of consciousness
25. Fainting
26. Tiredness upon awakening in the morning
27. Tiredness that prevents eating
28. Motion sickness in car, plane, or ship
29. Slowness of the body in adjusting to new situations

The Body is Self-correcting

Can you see the body in a long-term view? Can you imagine the transformations and adaptations that have occurred over the thousands of years of mankind's development? The human body has evolved with a complex system of defense and corrective mechanisms, which require little aid from us to keep the body functioning well. The body naturally corrects and adjusts its conditions. When we have overworked and the brain and head are tired, we yawn. When our back and waist feel sore and stiff, we stretch. When we overwork our fingers, we rub them. When our head aches, we press it. The human body works by the harmonization of various movements. Shiatsu, too, always strives to maintain harmony. When our body fails to work properly, we seek the help of a stronger hand to restore health. Shiatsu fills this need. Shiatsu gives the body direction so that its innate power of adaptation will function.

Similarly when we sleep, our bodies correct themselves. Thus they shift and move around. Through a person's posture during sleep, their condition may be diagnosed.

3. Techniques of Barefoot Shiatsu

Touch Techniques

The human body responds to three types of stimuli. When struck by some object it has a pain response. When exposed to heat or cold it has a thermal response. When touched in some manner the body has a tactile response. These three responses can be employed in treatment. Acupuncture uses the first type in the hope of producing a response to an object. Moxibustion employs the second type in its use of heat to produce changes in the body. Shiatsu and massage use the stimulus of touch pressure to alter energy flow within the body. Various types of pressure techniques are employed in shiatsu. It is important to remember that pressure is applied not merely with the fingertips, but with the weight of the entire body. We lean our body weight into each movement. In this manner, we use the whole body to bring about a total cure. Mere fingertip pressure causes pain and is of little benefit to the receiver.

Rubbing

Perhaps the most familiar form of touch technique is rubbing. When we are cold we rub the palms of our hands together. As it stimulates blood flow, rubbing is used to relieve fatigue and to improve the tone of the skin and muscles. When rubbing a patient, it is most important to remember to place the hands flat on the body and to maintain a steady pressure from the beginning to the end of the motion (Fig. 19).

Fig. 19

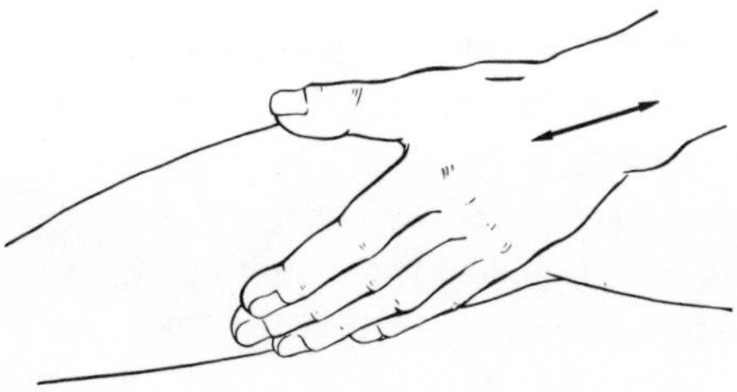

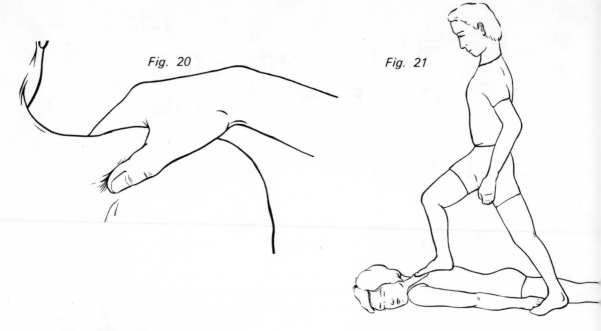

Fig. 20   Fig. 21

Kneading

Using the thumb alone or the thumb and index finger together, knead such areas as the tendons near joints, for example the elbow or knee. This pressure can also be applied along the back or sides of the neck and along the tops of the shoulders held in a "squeeze position." This motion loosens stiffness and increases ki flow in the area (Fig. 20).

Leaning into It (Pressing)

This technique is the one most frequently used in our shiatsu treatment. With the palm of the hand, the sole of the foot or the thumbs and fingers, the whole body leans into each movement. Allow this natural pressure to effect the desired results. Constant attention to body position and pressure will be very rewarding. All movement and pressure should originate from the *hara*. In other words do not merely press with the fingertips alone (See Fig. 21).

Tapping

Attention must be given to both speed and lightness in the tapping motion. It is important to tap lightly, quickly and rhythmically. Light tapping restores vitality to tired muscles and nerves, whereas excessively heavy striking could have an adverse effect on the muscles and nerves. Tapping is carried out with one or more fingers, with the palm, with the side or back of the hand, or with the fist (Fig. 22).

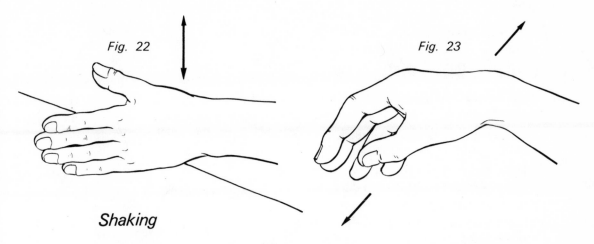

Fig. 22

Fig. 23

Shaking

The shaking movement can be administered by the receiver to himself or by the giver to the receiver. In the first case, with the whole body relaxed, the receiver vigorously shakes his hands or feet (Fig. 23). The shaking motion is used when there is a lack of vital energy, especially in the extremities. In the second case, the giver administers shaking to the receiver at the beginning of the shiatsu session. With a foot on the hip of the receiver, the giver gently shakes the entire body, thus relaxing the receiver and preparing him to receive deep shiatsu treatment.

Vibrating

Placing the palms or the fingers firmly on the receiver's skin and exerting a rapid to-and-fro motion, send a vibrating motion into the receiver. This vibration can be used effectively on the *hara* and on the eyes (with

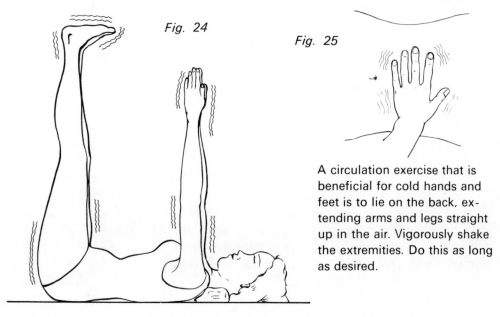

Fig. 24

Fig. 25

A circulation exercise that is beneficial for cold hands and feet is to lie on the back, extending arms and legs straight up in the air. Vigorously shake the extremities. Do this as long as desired.

very light pressure). Rhythmical vibration is effective in relieving numbness caused by weak muscles.

Moving (Stretching)

This technique is used to stretch the muscles and tendons of the leg and knee, arm and elbow areas. To stimulate a pressure point (*tsubo*) effectively, the muscle through which the meridian —pathway of energy—passes must be relaxed and receptive.

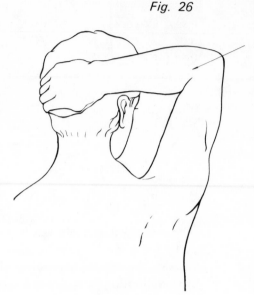

Fig. 26

Diagnosis

Generally, shiatsu is given as a preventative. Common sense tells us that it is much easier to stop a problem developing at the beginning than it is to cure it at an advanced stage. If the causes of illness are removed, the need for special curative treatment is eliminated. Regular shiatsu sessions will keep the ki flow circulating smoothly without congestion or stagnation. From time to time, however, conditions beyond our control arise and interrupt this smooth flow of energy. Extreme environmental conditions, such as heat or cold, excessive wind, poor quality food or irregular eating patterns, lack of sleep, and so forth, alter this biological energy flow. Mental stress and extreme pressure and tension from business or family life can also change the body's ability to receive and to discharge. In other words a condition can arise of disequilibrium or unequal exchange. When input is greater than output, we say excess exists; when output is greater than input, we say a deficiency exists. When problems do arise, the ability to correct symptoms depends on diagnostic ability. With correct diagnosis one can understand the primary cause of the disorder and alter it, thereby eliminating both the symptom and, more important, the cause. To remove only the symptom is partial treatment and a waste of time.

Diagnosis and treatment are one and the same. Without the ability to diagnose accurately, shiatsu therapy is merely recreation. For thousands of years, ancient healers of the Orient have been aware of an antagonistic yet complementary relationship in the body. Just as day has its opposite in night and man has his opposite in woman, this complementary antagonism exists in the body. Internal conditions are revealed on the outside of the body; for example, congested kidneys are manifested by abnormal conditions in the area beneath the eye. It is also true that external conditions (like cold winds) affect the internal condition (of the lungs in this case). These relationships can be very useful in making accurate, practical diagnoses.

The method of diagnosis by seeing is called *Bō-Shin*, or "diagnosis by observation." In everyday encounters, the first impression we have when meeting a person tells us something about them. Do you sometimes find yourself thinking, "He seems to be a very nice person," or "I'm glad he left, when he was here, I felt very nervous"? With practice we can use our naturally observant attitude and begin to diagnose internal conditions as well as emotional and psychological tendencies.

Front Diagnosis

Suppose a patient comes to see you. At your first meeting you can begin front diagnosis. As the person walks across the room to greet you, you will gain the first general impression. You observe the height, weight, proportions and general constitution. Is the body compact and small with a broad face (yang), or is the body larger and more expanded with an elongated face (yin)? Look at the pupils. Are they dilated or constricted? Are there any observable serious physical conditions? What is your impression of the person's emotional and psychological condition?

The following is a list of psychological traits that reflect internal problems:

Fear .... Kidneys
Serious timidity .... Lungs
Laughing excessively ...... Heart
Anger or short temper .... Liver
Moodiness .... Stomach

Visual diagnosis of outstanding facial features provides valuable information. Wrinkles on the forehead and swollen or contracted lips indicate upset in the digestive system. A swollen nose tells us of the heart's activity. Bags or dark circles under the eyes indicate malfunctioning of the kidneys. Skin and facial color and texture tell of the patient's past.

Generally, facial color may be interpreted in the following ways. Red indicates that the heart is overworking. A yin condition (caused by an excessive intake of sugar, fruit, fruit juices, liquid, dairy products, and so on) causes capillaries to expand, thereby creating a reddened face. Yellow is an indication of problems in the pancreas, liver, and gallbladder. A dark or grayish color is associated with kidney trouble. White or a pale color indicates bad lungs. Many people with allergies have this color. A milky white color can be caused by milk, yogurt and cheeses, such as cottage cheese.

Eye diagnosis adds information about the patient's condition. Are the eyes bloodshot? If so, in what parts? More than three or four bloodshot lines indicate the beginning of problems. If the lines are in the upper one third of the eye white, the problem is in the upper one third of the body (head, neck, and lung region). Bloodshot lines in the center of the eye indicate problems in the center region of the body (spleen, stomach, liver, and gallbladder). Bloodshot lines in the lower eye white indicate problems in the lower region of the body (kidneys, bladder, intestines, and sex organs).

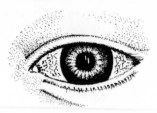

Fig. 27

As the person walks we should observe whether the movement is flexible or rigid. When the person reaches you and shakes hands, you can make a diagnosis from their hands. By feeling their temperature you can detect the activity of the heart. The hand should be slightly cool and dry. If it is cold, circulation is bad. If the hand is warm and feels sticky and oily, circulation is excessive, indicating that the heart is overworking because the person is taking in too much of such animal fats as butter or cheese. Rough skin confirms a diagnosis of excessive intake of animal food. The handshake also tells if the person trusts you or not. A firm handshake indicates trust; a limp one shows that the person is not yet willing to trust you.

As the person sits down, observe his breathing. Is the breath deep and smooth or is it shallow and fast? What is the odor of the breath and the odor of the body in general? Does the sound made of breathing indicate congestion in the sinus, bronchi, or lungs? This is *Bun-Shin* or "diagnosis through sound." As the person speaks you can begin to formulate your interpretation of his condition by the sound of his voice. Is it pleasant or rough? What does the person talk about? How does he express himself?

As you question the patient you are practicing *Mon-Shin*, "diagnosis by questioning." What is the main problem? At times the patient will be unable to tell you the true problem. You must develop an intuitive sense to see beyond the mere verbal description. With questioning you can find out the person's past. When was he born? Where did he grow up? What is his family situation? How many brothers and sisters does he have? In what type of occupation is he now or was he employed?

By the end of the conversation you have a very good idea of the person's past experiences, his present condition and of course his main symptomatic complaint. This overall view enables you to treat effectively. You now know the person's strong points and his weak points.

Next, the patient removes any jewelry, socks and stockings, and changes into a loose cotton gown in preparation for the shiatsu session. Light cotton clothing is best. As it is of vegetable origin, cotton will not interfere with the ki flow of the body. Synthetic clothing restricts the flow of ki and hurts the giver's fingers.

Side Diagnosis

While the receiver is standing, observing his overall condition from the side will confirm the tendencies observed from the front and will give additional information (Figs. 28 and 29).

A straight line from the top of the head to the feet should pass through the center of the ear and the center of the shoulder. Continuing down, this line should pass through the middle finger which is hanging

Fig. 28   Fig. 29

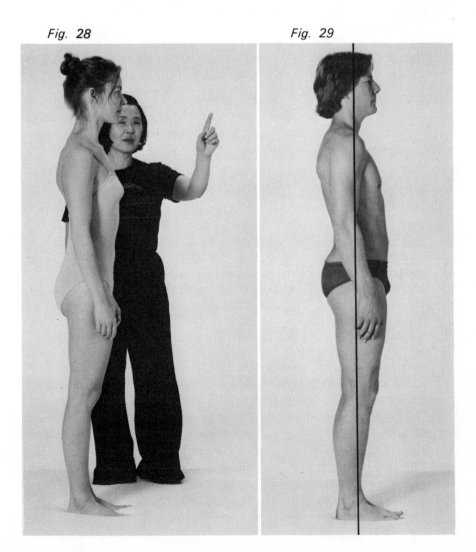

straight next to the leg. The body should appear relaxed. Neither leaning forward nor backward, but straight and comfortable is the natural posture.

The standing posture position is described as follows: 1. feet parallel about six inches apart; 2. head high, as if balancing a book; 3. chest out; 4. stomach and hips firm; 5. abdomen and back as flat as possible; 6. knees very lightly flexed, not stiffly locked; 7. weight evenly distributed between both feet, most of it falling on the balls of the feet.

The chin should be pulled in slightly. A chin thrusting outward indicates a tired brain. A person with such a condition could be suffering from exhaustion. The brain itself could be expanded (a yin condition), probably from an excessive intake of sugar, coffee, spices, drugs, fruit juices, and so on (yin foods). The forward-thrusting chin could indicate myopia or a lower region problem (for example, trouble in the pelvis).

The shoulders should be held straight in line with the center of the ear. Forward-drooping shoulders suggest lung or back problems or a spine that is out of alignment. If both shoulders are drawn tightly upward, it suggests liver problems, overeating, and intestinal difficulties.

The muscles in the front of the body—for example, the muscles in the area from the chest to the abdomen or on the inside of the arm or the back of the legs—shrink easily. This shrinkage causes them to tighten and harden, which thus affects the posture.

The stomach and the abdominal region should be flat. A stomach that sticks out or hangs down loosely, like a "beer belly," indicates the stomach and intestines are in an expanded (yin) condition. If there is an expansion under the ribs on the left side, the stomach is expanded.

Fig. 30 Postures

1. Correct posture.
2. Posture is all right. He stands straight, but his abdomen protrudes, indicating expanded stomach and liver.
3. Her body is held in a forward-leaning posture. Her lower abdomen protrudes. The shoulders are pulled in, weakening the digestive system.
4. The position of the upper body is all right, but the hips protrude too much, suggesting sex-organ problems.
5. He assumes a tired, listless posture. His chin protrudes, the shoulders are retracted, and the abdomen protrudes; consequently the neck cannot be held straight. Many older people have this condition.
6. His back is rounded, and his abdomen thrusts outward, indicating stomach and kidney problems.
7. This man has an extremely expanded abdomen, which suggests constipation and flatulence. He often has back problems and is excessively fat.

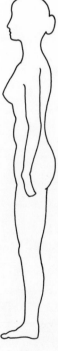

1

Rounded shoulders and curvature of the spine, both producing a roundness in the back, indicate expanded intestines and lung problems.

The center of gravity should be between the feet. The heels should be even when viewed from the rear. Balance placed rearward suggests expanded kidneys which drop the body's balance and move it backward. The balance should be on the balls of the feet. The head should hang forward very slightly, and with the eyes should be focused straight into the distance.

In females, a pelvis that rolls forward with attention drawn to the buttocks area indicates a crooked uterus.

Proper hip alignment is determined by the angle between the sacrum and the lumbar vertebrae. In males, proper hip alignment should be at 25 degrees, for females, it should be 30 degrees.

Fig. 31

Lumbar vertebrae

30°

Man 28°

Woman 30°

Sacrum

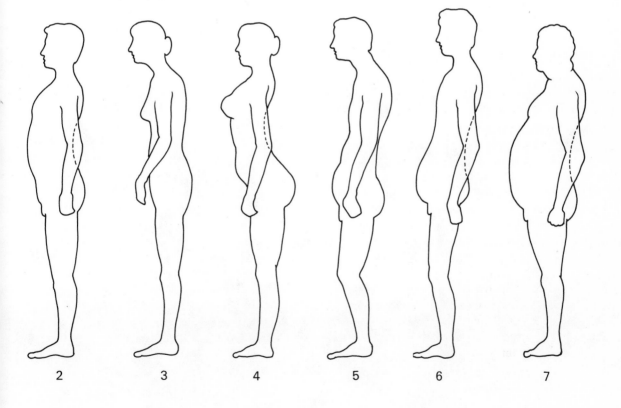

2   3   4   5   6   7

Back Diagnosis

Standing to the rear of the receiver, perform back diagnosis. Seen from the rear, the head of a healthy person should be straight, leaning neither to the left nor to the right. The shoulders should be level, neither held stiffly nor drooping. The arms should hang straight from the shoulders comfortably, without tension or curvature. The back should be flat with no expanded areas. The heels should be together; neither one should be in a forward or backward position. The hips should be level, and neither right nor left side should protrude (Figs. 32 and 33).

A head tilted to one side indicates an imbalance in the right and left sides of the body.

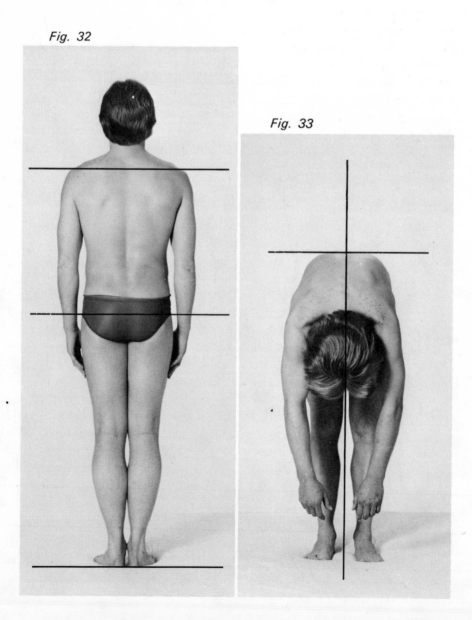

Fig. 32

Fig. 33

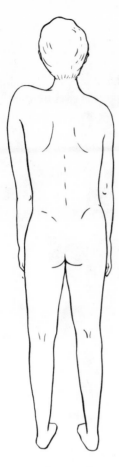

Fig. 34

See if the shoulders are level. A high right
shoulder indicates an imbalance between the
right and left sides of the body. There is an
expanding force on the right side, which pushes
up the right shoulder.

Consider the cause of this expansion. Is it an
expanded right lung, an enlarged and swollen
liver or perhaps congestion in the intestines on
the right side of the body? If the left shoulder is
raised, we know that there is an expansion on
the left side. It could be an expanded stomach,
problems in the spleen and pancreas, an expanded
left lung, bone problems or perhaps stagnation in
the intestines on the left side.

The arms are related to the brain. If they do not hang straight from
the shoulders, this could indicate nervous problems. Tightness is manifested as an inward curving of the arms, a position a person carrying
books might assume (see Figs. 30, No. 3).

An expansion or bulge over the lung or kidney region indicates either
expansion or congestion of those organs. Usually, if the person is eating
animal food with a high saturated fat content (hamburger, pork chops,
cheese, butter, and so on), mucous deposits will accumulate in the organ
and cause congestion.

Have the patient, who is now dressed in a loose cotton shirt or gown,
move into the area you have designated for the shiatsu session. The
room should be clean and comfortable. A quiet area is best in order to
relax the receiver, thereby increasing his receptivity to the treatment. The
treatment will take place on the floor. No special table or other equipment is necessary, though a carpeted floor spread with a towel or blanket
ensures the comfort of the receiver. Mats or cushions are fine. The point
is that nothing special is needed, but the comfort of the receiver should
always be considered.

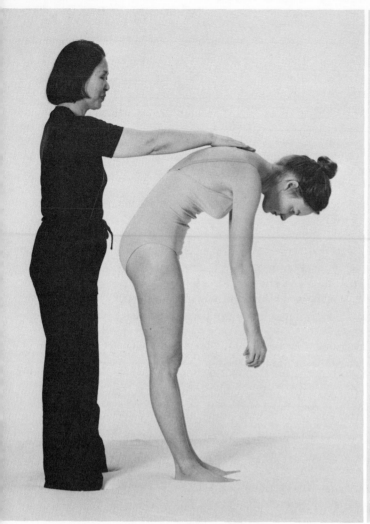
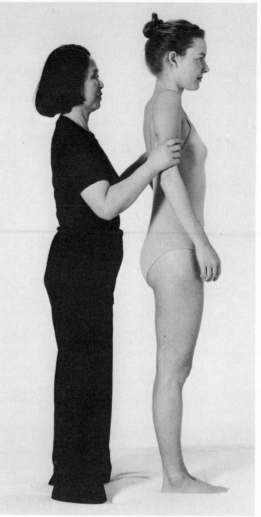

Fig. 35   Fig. 36

Have the patient bend forward, as you observe the spine. "Diagnosis through touch" is called *Setsu-Shin*. Place your hand on the vertebrae, beginning at the neck. Notice any subluxations (pushed-in vertebrae) or protrusions (pushed-out vertebrae). Is the spine straight? Feel each vertebra. Be attentive to any distortion, twists or pulling to the left or the right (Fig. 35).

Standing behind the receiver, grip both upper arms. Lift the arms up and down. This will give you information on the type of treatment you must give. The upper arms and upper thighs are related. Both indicate the overall nourishment of the body. If the arms are very large and flabby, the patient is overnourished. The muscle condition of the body can be examined in this area. If the skin texture is rough or if redness, soreness, or pimples are present, the person may have been, or may be, consuming an excess of animal food. If the arms and shoulders are very tight and stiff, this suggests tension in the body. This person is a nervous type. There are many meridians that pass through the upper arm-shoulder area. Trouble in the flow of energy within any of the meridians will be reflected in the upper arm (Fig. 36).

Stand back to back. The giver hooks her arms in the arms of the receiver. The giver spreads her legs, keeping the balance low, then, with knees bent, gently draws the receiver up on her back. Gravity does the work. The patient's hip is above that of the giver. In this position one can ask the following diagnostic questions: What is the overall flexibility? Is the receiver's body stiff and rigid or firm yet relaxed? Estimate the body weight. Is the body heavy or light? Does the body seem watery and expanded or is it tight and compact? Placing a body on the back reveals both the patient's overall flexibility and the condition of the kidney and bladder systems. If the balance is kept low, and concentration is held on the one point in *hara*, extremely heavy persons may be lifted without strain (Fig. 37).

Fig. 37

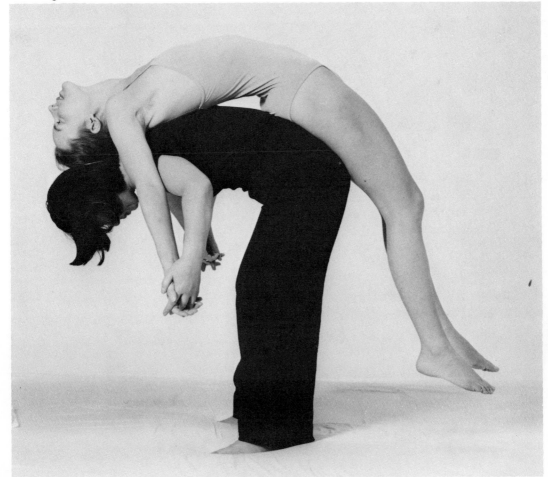

Full Body Treatment

Back Side

1. Have the receiver assume a seated position. Japanese style, *seiza*, is very good, but any posture with the back straight is fine. Tightness and stiffness in the shoulders indicates that the digestive system is not healthy. Kneeling behind the receiver, gently loosen the shoulders and neck with massage. Knead and relax the shoulders from the center toward the outside.

Kneeling on the left side of the receiver, find the medulla oblongata, or the hollow in the center at the base of the skull. Place your left thumb and forefinger on the temples. Place your right thumb on the medulla oblongata. Gently rock the head back onto the thumb and hold for three seconds (Figs. 38 and 39).

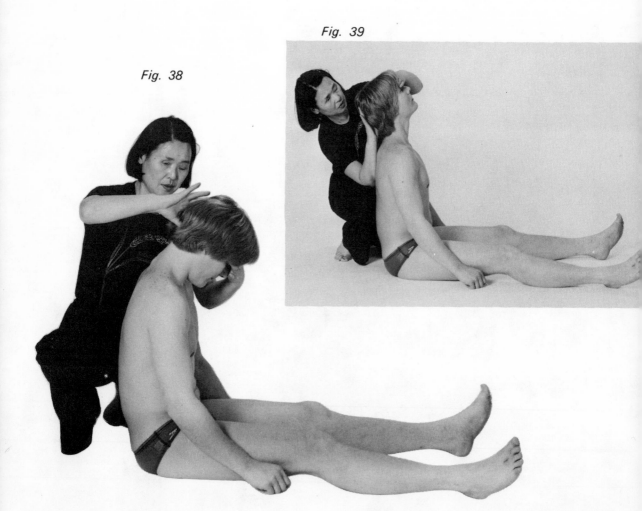

Fig. 39

Fig. 38

Move the right thumb to the left. There is another hollow about three inches from the center. Stimulate as before. This affects the autonomic nervous system (Fig. 40).

Change sides. Kneel on the right side of the receiver. Place your right thumb and forefinger on the temples. Place your left thumb in the hollow about three inches to the right of the medulla oblongata. Rock the head back onto the thumb. Hold for three seconds.

2. Have the receiver lie face down on the floor, with toes turned in and arms straight out at a ninety degree-angle to the rest of the body.

3. Stand to the side, at the waist, and roll the pelvis with the right foot (Fig. 41). When you feel that the receiver is relaxed you may proceed.

Fig. **41**

Fig. **40**

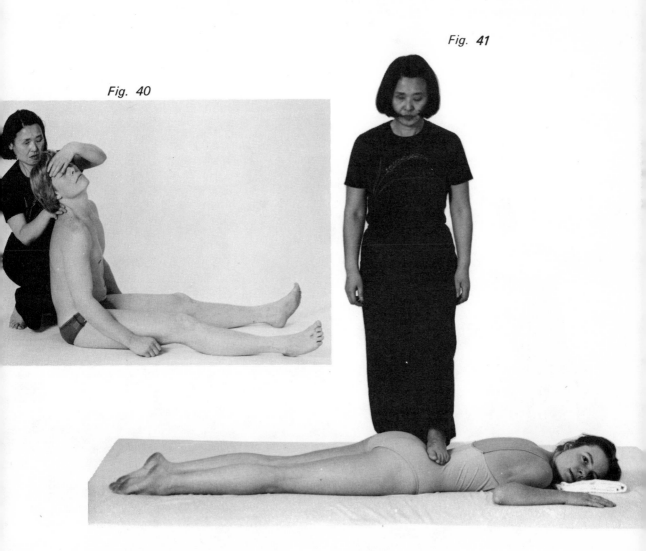

74

Fig. 42

Fig. 43

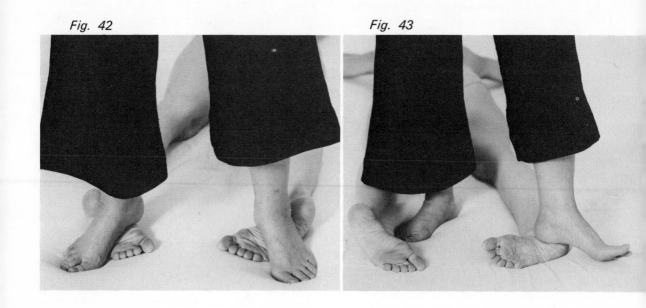

Fig. 44

Fig. 45

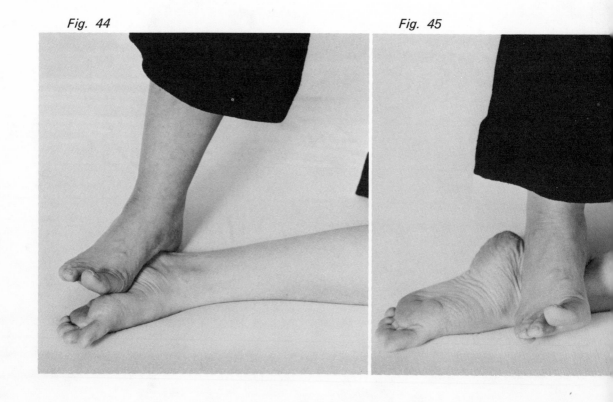

4. Standing between the receiver's feet, facing away from the body, gently walk up on the bottoms of the feet (Fig. 42). Walk from the heel toward the toes. Take care not to put all your weight on the toes. Walking on both feet simultaneously, shift your weight from one side to the other. You may walk on the feet for as long as you and the receiver feel comfortable. You can press your own feet by standing on a rolling pin.

5. Remain standing between the receiver's legs and press out the ankles (Fig. 43). With your left foot press down gently on the receiver's right ankle. Change feet and press down on the receiver's left ankle. Slowly stretch the muscles of the ankles.

6. Stand to the left side of the receiver. With your left foot press down and outward on the Achilles' tendon. Then, starting close to the heel, with your right foot lean your weight into the leg muscle, moving up the leg to below the knee (Figs. 44 to 46). Never press on the knee!

Fig. 46

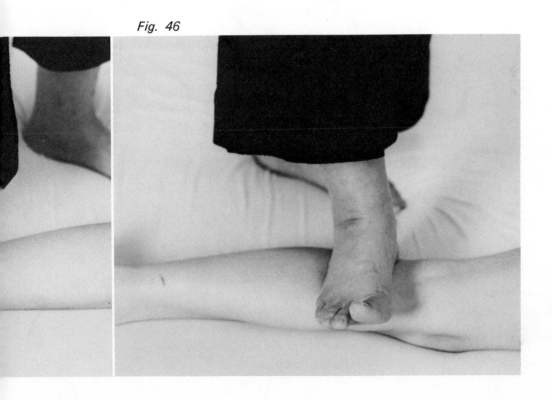

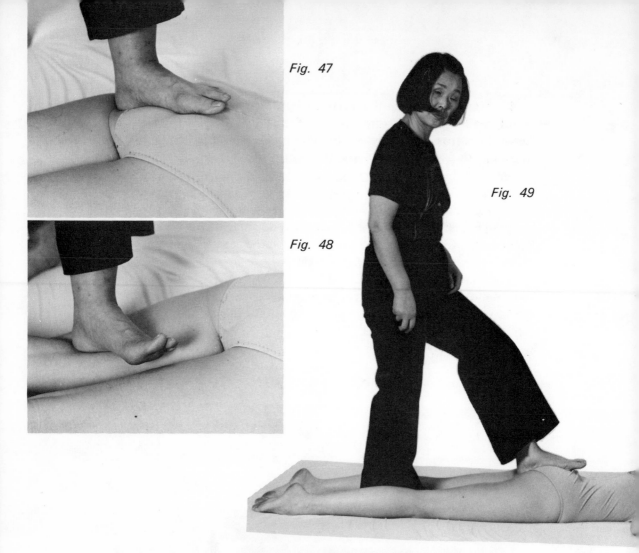

Fig. 47

Fig. 49

Fig. 48

7. In order to use your energy economically, always employ your closest hand or foot to treat the receiver. You should always make use of the right position. Change feet and, with the left foot, stimulate the left thigh. With the heel resting on the leg, lean your body weight on the upper leg region, working down the outside of the leg to the top of the knee (Figs. 47 and 48). Work down the middle of the upper thigh to the top of the knee. Repeat. While using your foot you should feel the muscle and bone; you are not just pressing. You must be sensitive with your foot.

8. Move to the receiver's right side. With your left foot press down and outward on the Achilles' tendon. Start close to the heel. With your left foot lean your weight into the leg muscle moving up the leg to below the knee.

9. Change feet and with the right foot stimulate the right thigh. With the heel resting on the leg, lean your body weight on the upper leg region, working down the outside and then the center of the thigh. Repeat.

10. Stand between the receiver's legs, facing toward the head. Place your foot on the tailbone, or coccyx, and lean your weight into this area three times (Figs. 49 and 50). The stimulation should go from the tailbone up the spinal column toward the head. Step along the inside of the thighs, moving down to the top of the knee and back around in a horseshoe shape. The lumbo-sacral plexus and the sciatic nerve are located in this area. Stimulation of the tailbone relaxes the autonomic nervous system. Stimulate this area slowly and deeply. You will be surprised at how the body will begin to relax.

11. Gripping a chair, stand on the upper legs (Fig. 51). Shift your weight from side to side as you walk down the legs.

Fig. 50

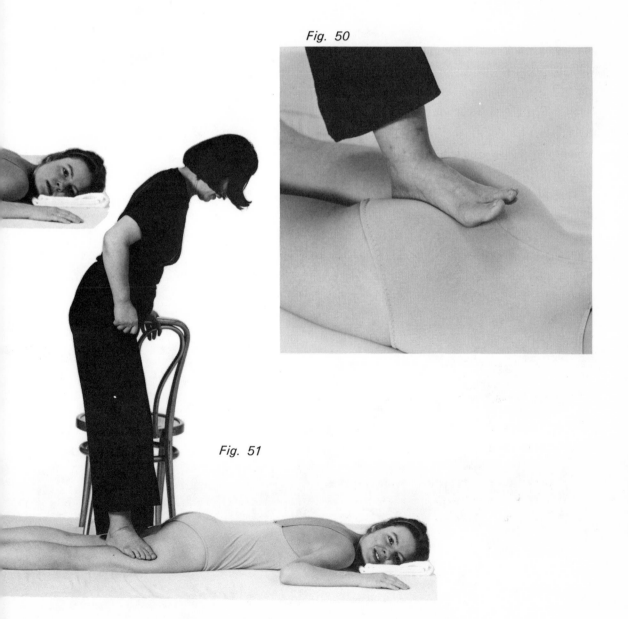

Fig. 51

12.   Stand behind the receiver's right arm. Placing your right foot on the outstretched hand, which is placed palm down, lean your entire weight on the outstretched hand. Always use the closest foot (Fig. 52). Step from the back of the hand down the fingers. Stimulating the hand first will allow the entire arm to relax and to open up to further stimulation.

13.   Change feet and use your left foot. Lean your weight on the upper arm and the shoulder above the biceps (Fig. 53). Proceed downward to the elbow. Do not walk on the elbow! Pass over the elbow and resume leaning your weight on the forearm (Fig. 54).

14.   Change to the left side of the receiver's body. Stand behind the left arm. Lean your weight on the outstretched hand, palm down, with the left foot.

Fig. 52

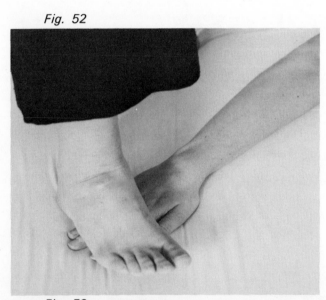

Fig. 53

Fig. 54

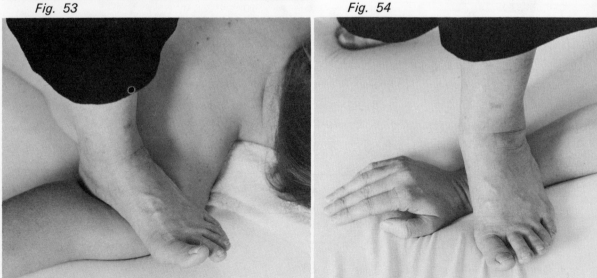

15. Change feet. Use the right foot to lean into the shoulder and work down the upper arm to the elbow. Avoid the elbow! Continue stimulation of the forearm.

16. The practitioner can use the palms of the hands to press the back. Go down the center on the spine (Fig. 55). Always lean your body weight on the back.

17. Only if the practitioner has confidence should be perform this technique. Step up on the buttocks near the waist with most of your weight (Fig. 56). A chair can be used for balance. With one foot near the waist bone use the other foot to press gently and loosen the back.

Fig. 55

Fig. 56

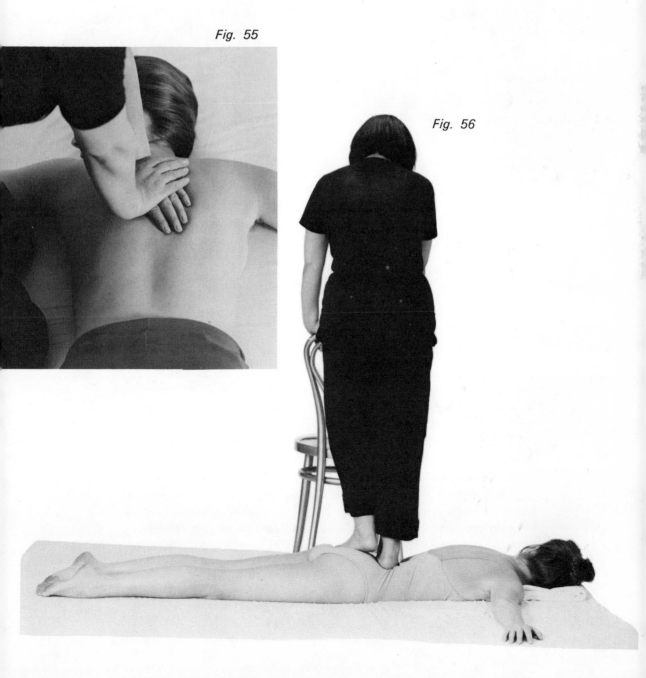

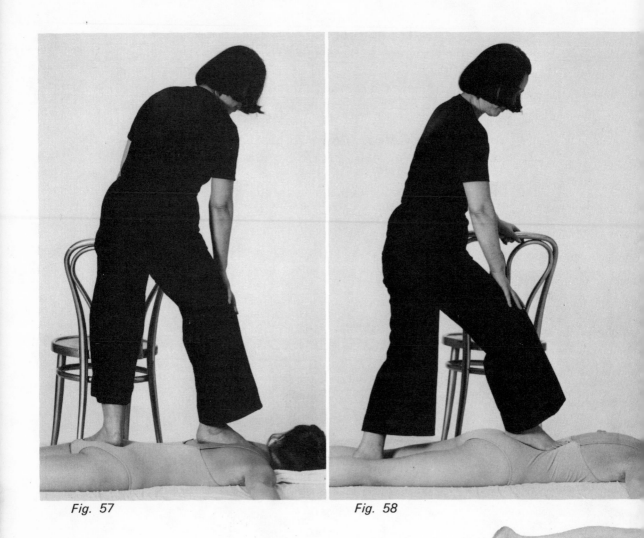

Fig. 57   Fig. 58

18.   Press the spine from the neck downward (Figs. 57 and 58).
Remember that most of the giver's body weight remains on the hipbone and the pressure exerted on the body is always controlled and
distributed according to the receiver's condition.

This type of stimulation can be done by either standing directly on
the body or by standing to the side of the body (Fig. 59).

19.   Stand with feet astride the receiver and knead the shoulders
(Fig. 60). The body position assumes a triangular shape when working
down the bladder meridian of the back. Unconscious attention comes
from the *hara* and the head, while conscious attention is in the hands.
Balance is maintained with this interaction of *hara*, head and hands.

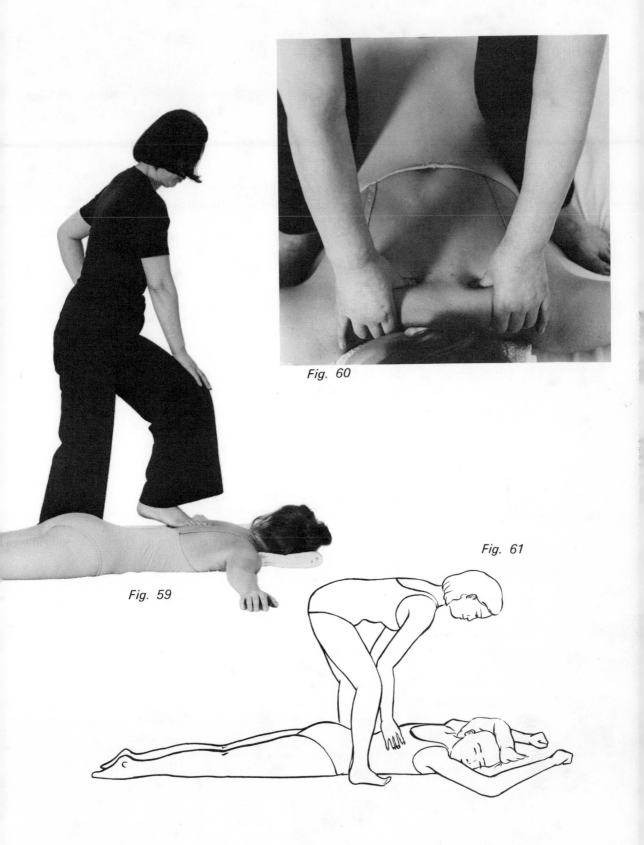

Fig. 60

Fig. 59

Fig. 61

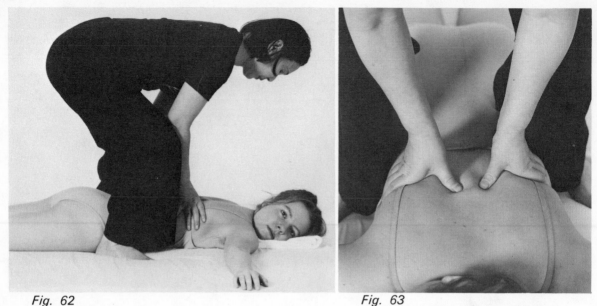

Fig. 62   Fig. 63

Using the thumbs, stimulate the inner bladder meridian. Beginning at the seventh cervical vertebra—the large knob-like projection at the base of the neck—place the thumbs about one-and-one-half-inches away from each side of the spinal column (Figs. 62 and 63). Synchronize your breathing with the receiver's by telling him to "Breathe in . . . . Breath out." Both giver and receiver should breathe at the same time. On the exhalation, lean into the receiver's back. Hold for five to seven seconds. Allow gravity to do the work. Keeping your back as straight as possible, simply bend your knees and allow natural weight to give the pressure. Weight concentration is on the thumb joint, not on the tip. Relax; do not exert strong pressure. Coordinated breathing and natural body weight are all that are necessary to give a very effective stimulation to this important area. Concentration and balance come from the triangle formed by the *hara*, the hands and the head. These bladder meridian points are also called *Yu* points, the points where energy and life force enter the body. Stimulation of this region energizes and harmonizes the entire body.

We can diagnose the condition of the internal organs by sensitivity, pain or hardness felt along this meridian channel.

Proceed down the back at one-and-one-half-to two-inches intervals. Always coordinate your breathing with your patient's. Stop at the tail-bone area. Repeat.

20.   Return to the neck region. Place thumbs about one-and-one-half-inches on either side of the first bladder line. This second bladder line runs from the edge of the shoulder blade, or scapula, down the length of the back to the coccyx.

Fig. 64   Spinal Diagnosis

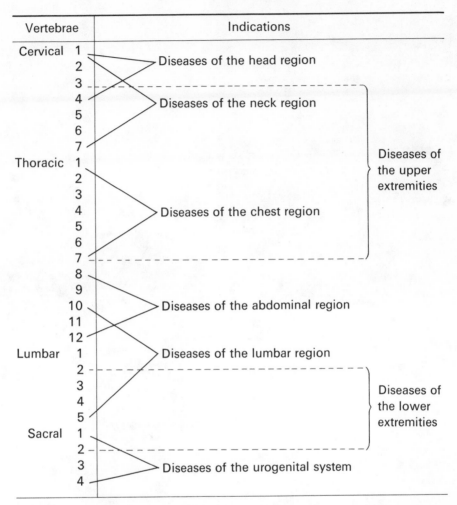

Vertebrae	Indications
Cervical 1 2 3 4 5 6 7	Diseases of the head region Diseases of the neck region
Thoracic 1 2 3 4 5 6 7	Diseases of the chest region Diseases of the upper extremities
8 9 10 11 12	Diseases of the abdominal region
Lumbar 1 2 3 4 5	Diseases of the lumbar region Diseases of the lower extremities
Sacral 1 2 3 4	Diseases of the urogenital system

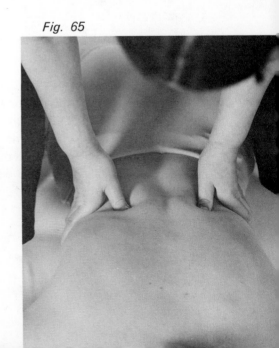

Fig. 65

Coordinate your breathing with your patient's. On the exhalation, lean your weight into the back. Hold for five to seven seconds. Move downward at one-and-one-half-to two-inches intervals, keeping the knees bent and allowing natural body pressure to stimulate the points (Fig. 65). Relax. Natural body pressure acts like a child walking across your back. It is effortless. Stimulate this line once.

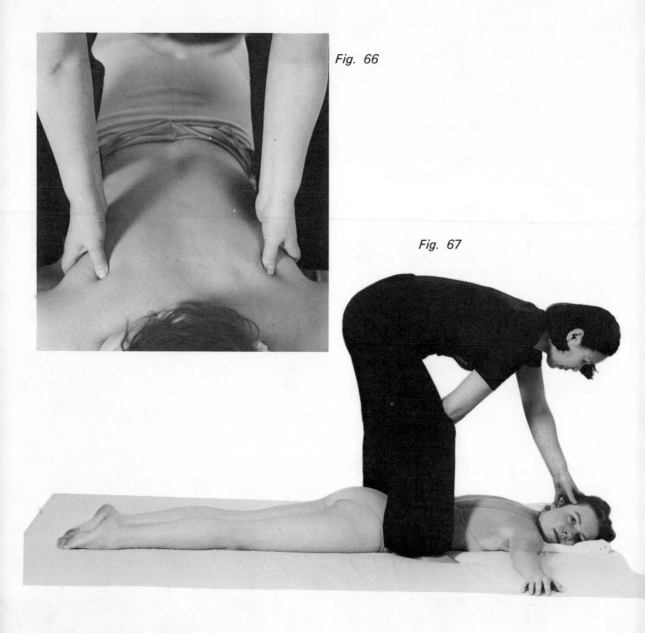

Fig. 66

Fig. 67

21. Place your thumbs on the upper back in the centers of the shoulder blades (Fig. 66). These points are on the small intestine meridian. Lean your body weight on these points and coordinate your breathing with your patient's. Proceed downward along the outer contour of the back stimulating at one-and-one-half-to two-inches intervals. Stop at the hip. The last point aids in the relief of constipation. Go down this third line once or twice.

22.   Stimulate the neck line (Fig. 67), the gallbladder meridian (around the ear and cheek as well as the side of the face), and the eye point (Figs. 68 and 69).

23.   Place your right hand at the receiver's left shoulder. With the left hand take the receiver's left wrist and lift it, stretching the arm (Fig. 70). Rotate it several times in both the clockwise and the counterclockwise direction.

Bend the arm at the elbow and place the receiver's hand as far up on the back as is comfortable (Fig. 71).

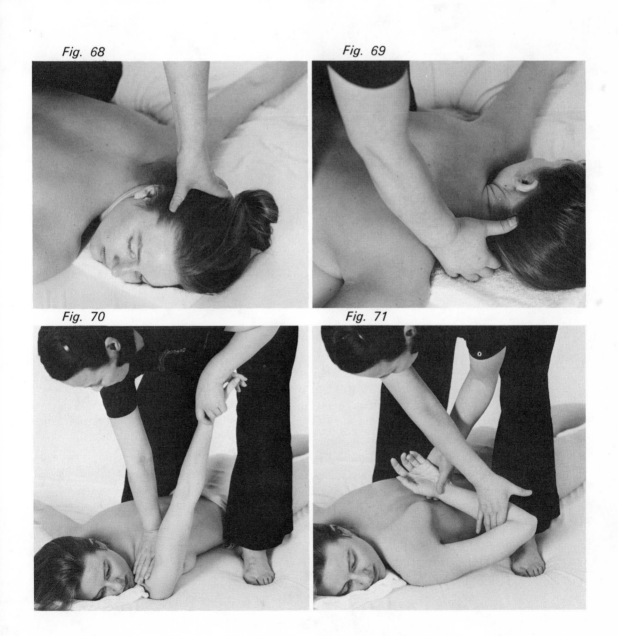

Fig. 68

Fig. 69

Fig. 70

Fig. 71

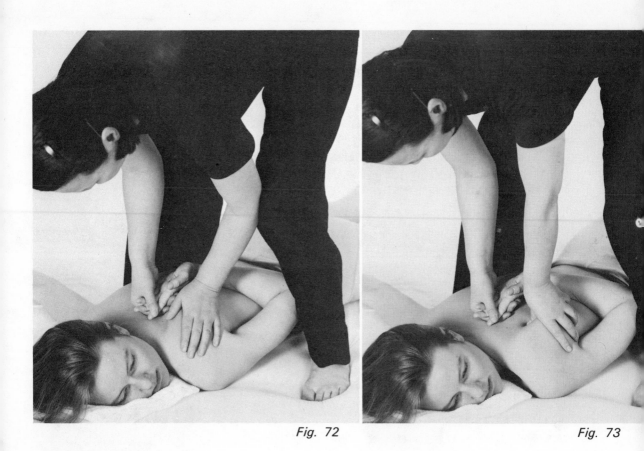

Fig. 72   Fig. 73

Change hands. Hold the receiver's left hand with your right hand.
With the left hand on the shoulder blade, lean your body weight on this
area and loosen any congestion that may be lodged under the shoulder
blade (Fig. 72). Follow the contour of the shoulder blade while pressing
(Fig. 73). Make an adjustment by pushing the arm upward toward the
back of the neck (Fig. 74).

24.   Change arms. Stimulate the right side. Place your left hand at
the shoulder. With the right hand pick up the receiver's right wrist and
lift and stretch the arm. Rotate it several times in each direction. Bend
the arm at the elbow and place the receiver's hand as far up on the
back as is comfortable. Hold the receiver's right hand with your left
hand. With your right hand on the shoulder blade, lean your body
weight on the blade and loosen it.

25.   Stretch the arms (Figs. 75 and 76).

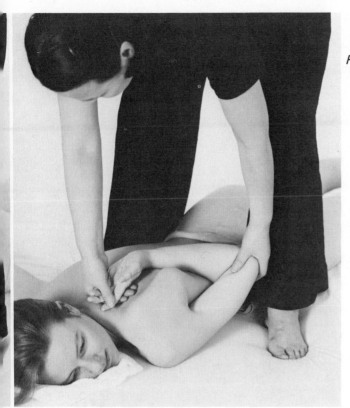

Fig. 74

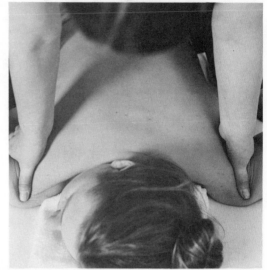

Fig. 75

Fig. 76

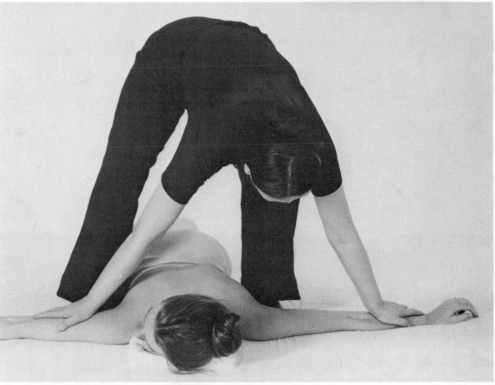

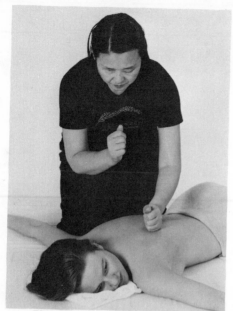

Fig. 77

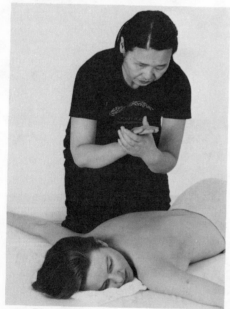

Fig. 78

Fig. 79

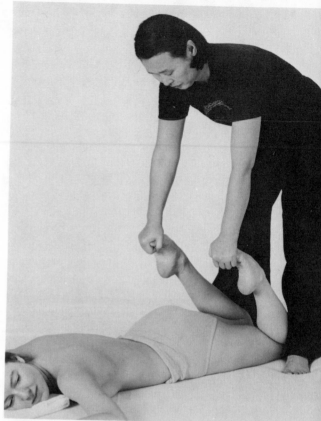

Fig. 80

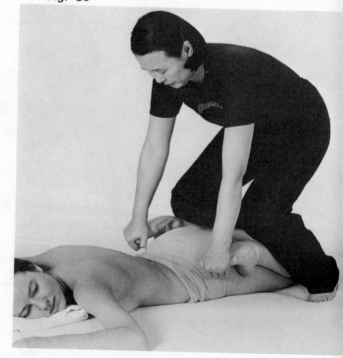

26.   Kneel to the side of the receiver. With lightly closed fists gently pound the back (Fig. 77). This pounding is very relaxing to the receiver, you can also pound by holding your hands palm to palm and lightly striking with the back of your hand (Fig. 78).

27.   Stand at the receiver's feet. Her knees are bent. Grip the toes and lean your body weight on the legs (Fig. 79), bending them into the receiver's back. Stretch the legs to the floor if possible (Fig. 80). Cross the ankles and lean the legs on the back again (Fig. 81). Reverse the ankles and repeat the downward stretch.

28.   Straighten the legs. Hold her left ankle. Place your right foot on the pelvis. Pull upward, diagonally, stretching the leg (Fig. 82). Return the leg to its resting position. Repeat this from the other side of the receiver.

Fig. 82

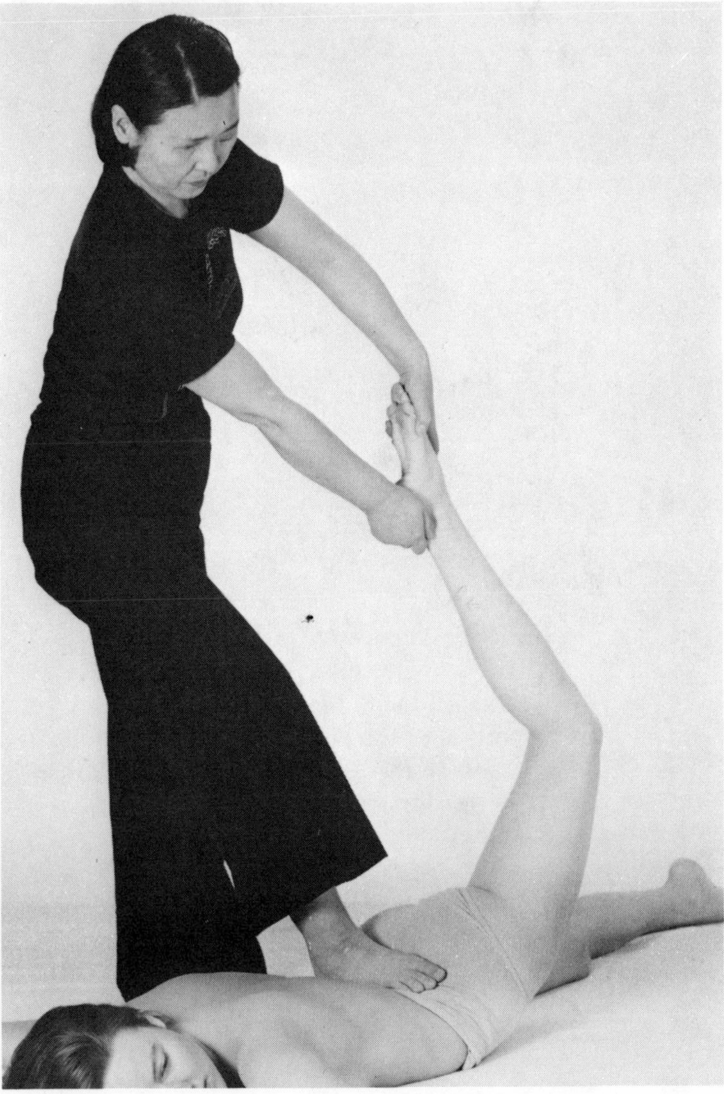

Fig. 81

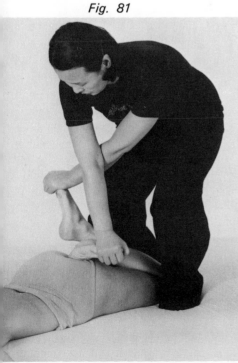

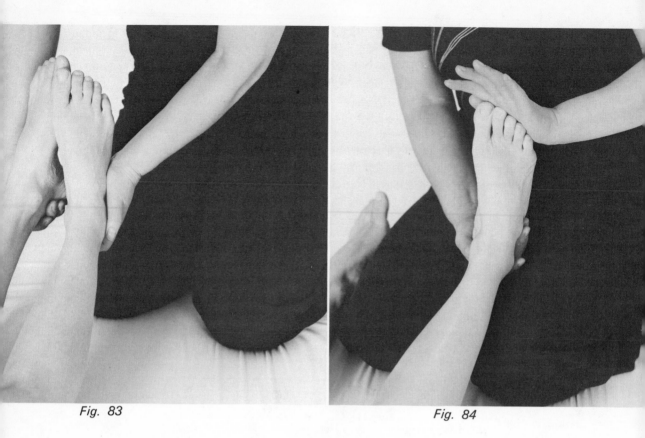

Fig. 83   Fig. 84

Front Side

29.   Have the receiver turn over on his back.

30.   Sit at the receiver's feet. Hold both legs and lift them three to four inches off the floor (Fig. 83). Sway back and forth, relaxing the lower portion of the body. Open the legs and drop the feet.

31.   Pick up the right foot. Hold it with your right hand. With your left hand brush the toes (Figs. 84 to 86). Their flexibility reveals the leg's condition. Stimulate the sides of each toe with the left hand (Fig. 87). Change hands. Hold the foot with your left hand. Turn the foot to the side and massage its bottom with the right thumb (Fig. 88).

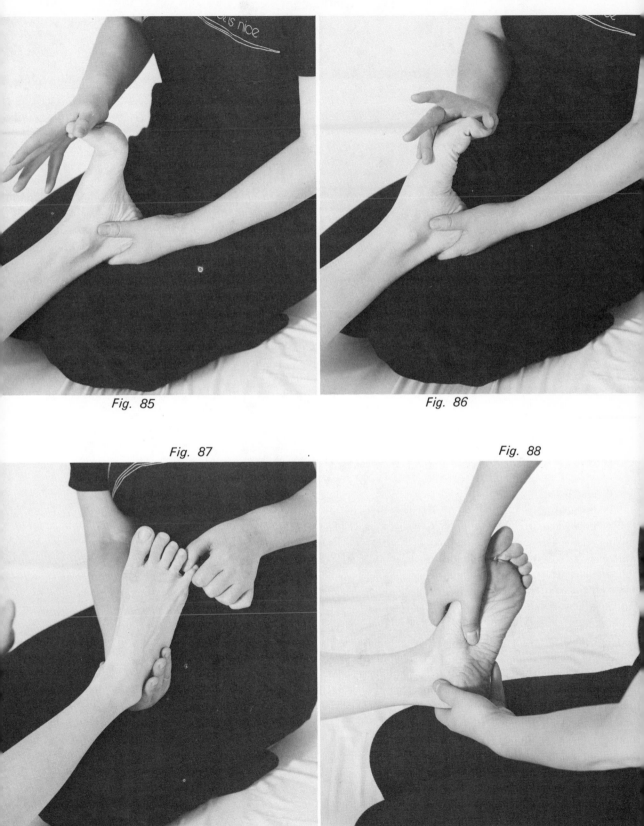

Fig. 85

Fig. 86

Fig. 87

Fig. 88

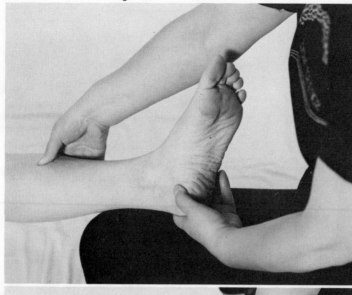

Fig. 89

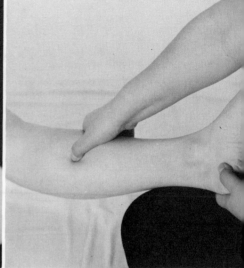

Fig. 90

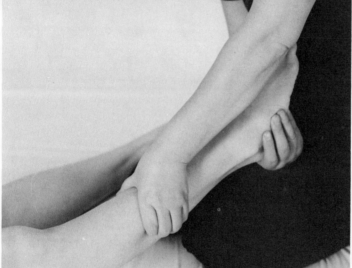

Fig. 91

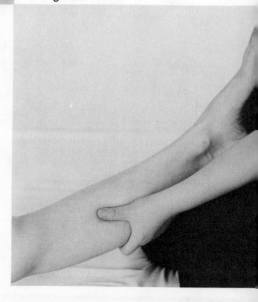

Fig. 92

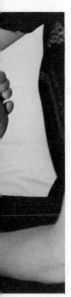

32.   Massage the top of the leg along the shinbone from the ankle to below the knee (Fig. 89). This stimulates the spleen meridian.

33.   With the right thumb massage up under the shinbone from the ankle to below the knee. About four fingers above the anklebone is the point related to sexual functions (Fig. 90).

34.   Change hands. Wrap four fingers of your right hand around the outside of the shinbone and massage upward (Fig. 91). This stimulates the gallbladder meridian.

35.   With the right thumb massage the calf muscle (Fig. 92). Pain in this area indicates congestion in the bladder meridian.

36.   Hold the heel with one hand. With your free hand rotate the ankle three times in each direction. Pull the heel toward you and drop the foot.

37.   Change feet. Pick up the left foot and hold the heel in your left palm. With your right hand brush the toes in a back-and-forth motion.

38.   Massage the top of the left leg from the ankle on the outside of the shinbone.

39.   Massage up under the shinbone from the ankle to below the knee with the right thumb.

40.   Wrap your four fingers around the outside of the shinbone and massage upward.

41.   Change hands. With the left hand massage the calf muscle.

42.   Three fingers below the kneecap on the outside of the leg on both legs is located the point called *Sanri*, or stomach meridian point No. 36 (Fig. 93). Press this point with the thumb three times for ten seconds each time.

Fig. 93

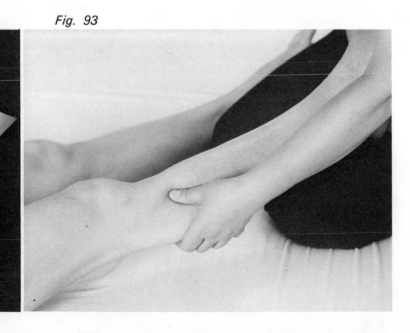

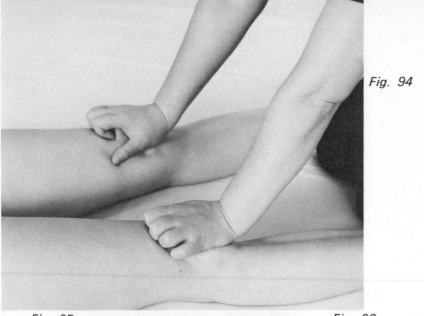

Fig. 94

Fig. 95   *Fig. 96*

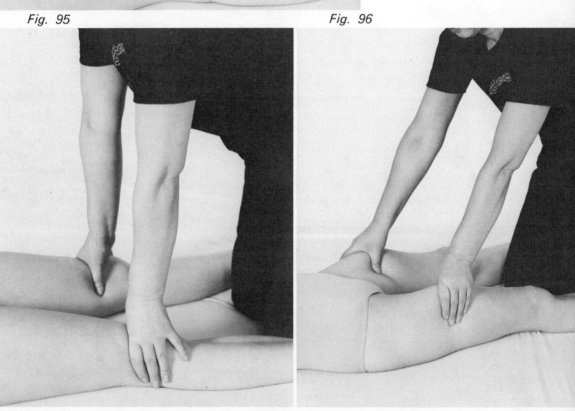

43.   Rotate the ankle in both directions. Holding the heel, pull it toward you and then drop the foot.

44.   Move between the receiver's legs. Place your open palms on kneecaps (Fig. 94). Put your weight on your palm and gently push up and down. Check the movement of the kneecap. Many meridians flow under the kneecap.

45. With your thumb and index finger spread apart, massage up the front of the leg from the top of the knee to the pelvis (Figs. 95 to 97). Lean into the leg with your entire body weight and squeeze. Massage both legs simultaneously.

46. Hold the receiver's right ankle with your left hand. Place your right hand on her right knee (Fig. 98). Bend the knee and stretch it. Push it down toward the chest (Fig. 99). Sometimes you can go deeper.

Fig. 97

Fig. 98

Fig. 99

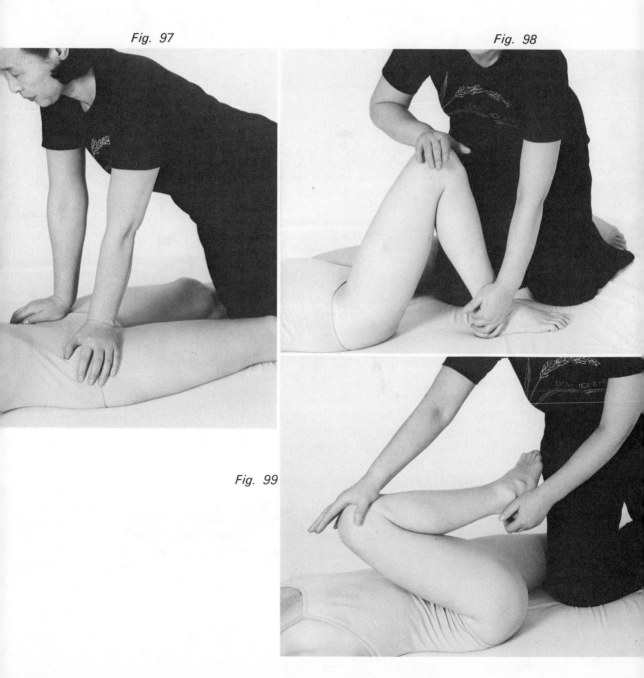

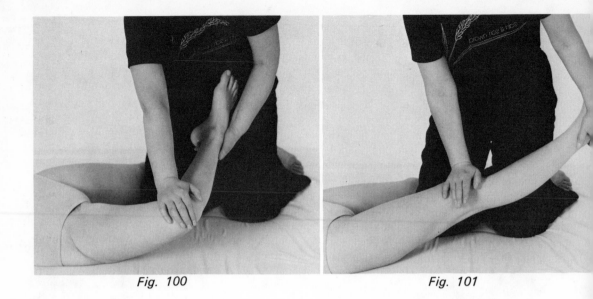

Fig. 100   Fig. 101

Rotate the knee outward, allowing the knee to go to the floor (Fig. 100).
Adjust and stretch the leg by pulling outward with the heel. Avoid exerting pressure on the kneecap. The hand is on the knee for guidance, not
for pressure.

If it suits the receiver's condition, push outward (Fig. 101).

Repeat all the procedures of step 46 on the left leg using the opposite
hands.

47.   Move to the receiver's right side. Kneel between the body and
the outstretched arm.

48.   Massage each finger individually (Fig. 102). With the receiver's
hand outstretched, massage from the small finger to the index finger
(Fig. 103). Change hands to massage the thumbs (Fig. 104). Knead the

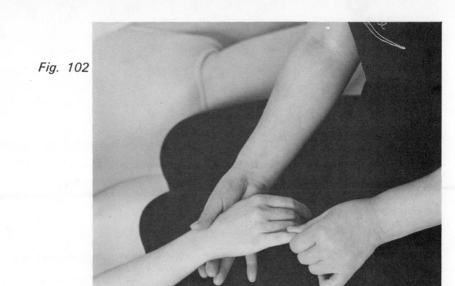

Fig. 102

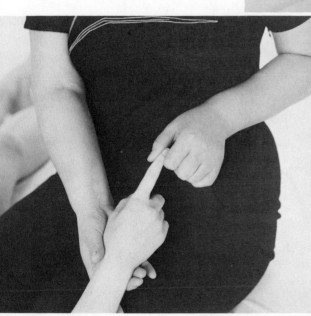

Fig. 103

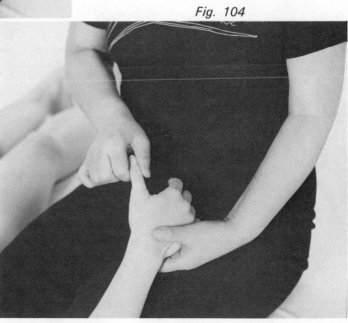

Fig. 104

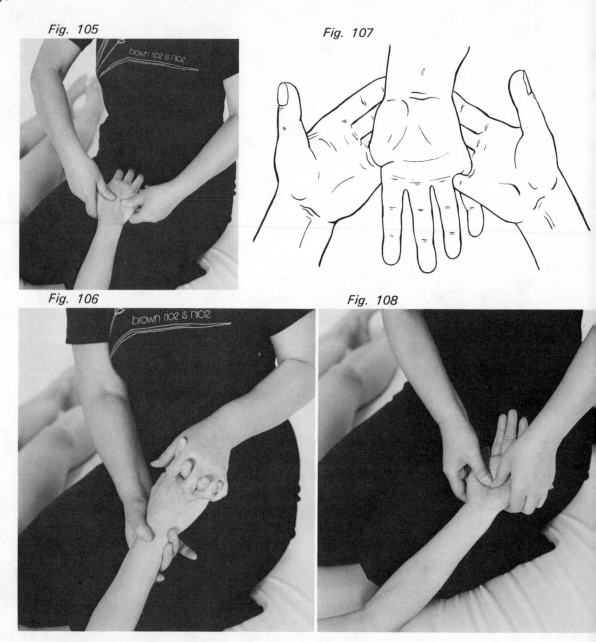

Fig. 105

Fig. 107

Fig. 106

Fig. 108

palm and press on the top of the hand (Fig. 105). Bend the wrist back toward the body stretching the fingers (Fig. 106).

Turn the palm up. Place the little finger of your right hand between your patient's little finger and ring finger. Place the little finger of your left hand between your patient's index finger and thumb. Spread and stretch the palm open (Fig. 107). Massage this palm area with your thumbs (Fig. 108).

49.   Hold your patient's hand with your right hand. With your left hand, beginning at the wrist, massage upward directly above the front of the index finger to the elbow (Figs. 109 and 110). Simultaneously stimulate the arm following the bone with the thumb and the back of the arm with the index finger. Massage this area twice. This will stimulate the large intestine meridian on the top of the arm and the heart meridian on the back of the arm.

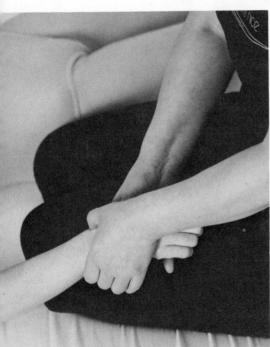

Fig. 109

Fig. 110

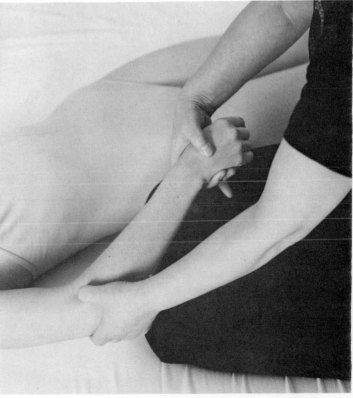

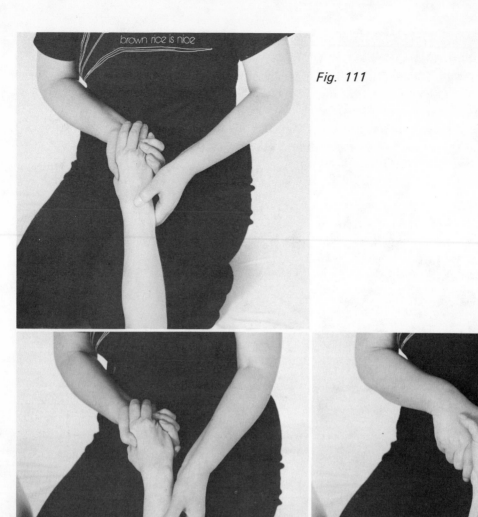

Fig. 111

Fig. 112

Fig. 113

Massage the middle of the arm to the elbow (Figs. 111 and 112). Again apply pressure to both the top and back of the arm. Massaging the top of the arm stimulates the triple-heater meridian, while massage to the back of the arm stimulates the heart governor meridian.

Turn the hand over. Massage up the center of the arm to the elbow (Fig. 113). The thumb stimulates the lung meridian while the index finger stimulates the small intestine meridian. Massage each line twice.

Fig. 114   Fig. 115

Fig. 116

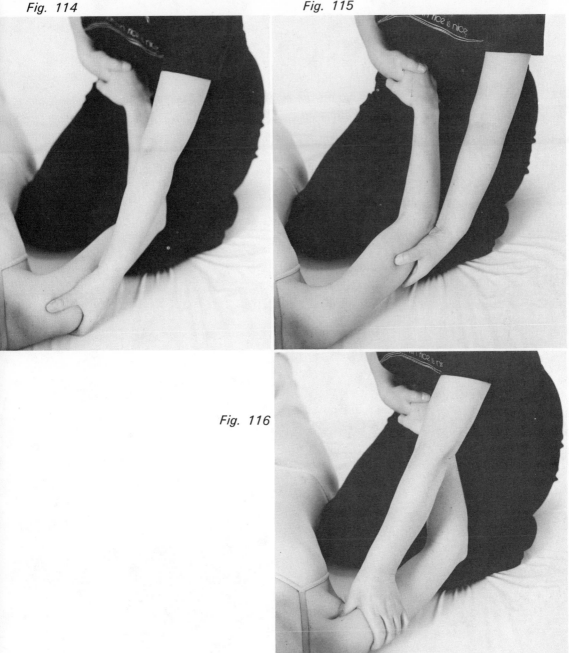

50.   Massage down the upper arm, from the shoulder to the elbow (Figs. 114 and 115). This time do not be concerned with meridians; just apply hand pressure while following the bone and muscle. Stimulate the center, the inside and the outside of the upper arm (Fig. 116).

Stimulate the elbow area well (Fig. 117). Adjust the arm by bending it and pulling the wrist outward (Figs. 118 and 119). Release the arm.

51.   Change your position to directly face the receiver's trunk area. Feel the liver under the rib cage on the right side of the body (Fig. 120). Feel the gallbladder and large intestines (Figs. 121 and 122).

Fig. 117

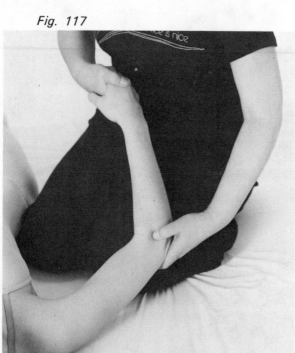

Fig. 118

Fig. 119

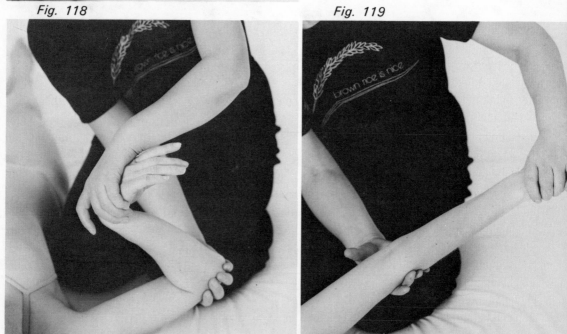

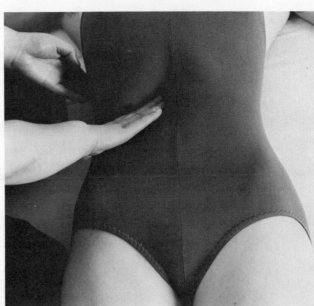

Fig. 120

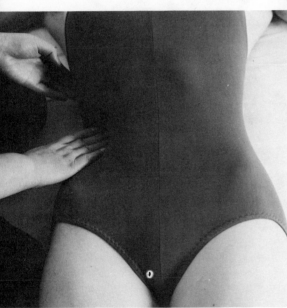

Fig. 121

Fig. 122

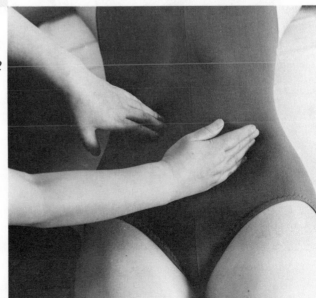

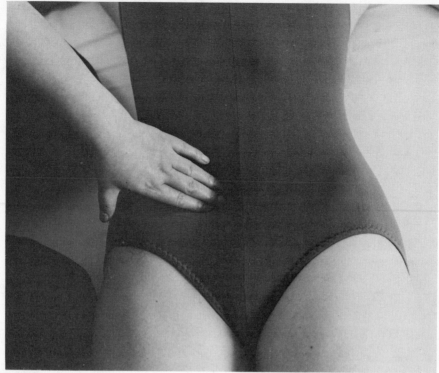

Fig. 123

Fig. 124   Internal Organs

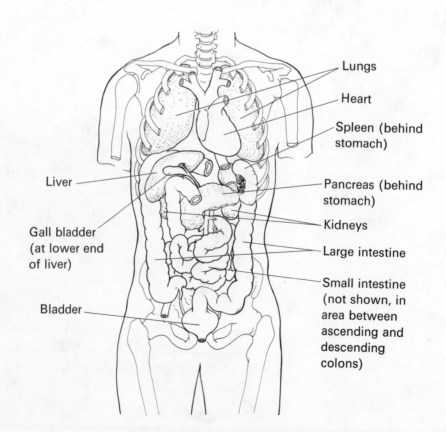

Lungs

Heart

Spleen (behind
stomach)

Liver

Pancreas (behind
stomach)

Kidneys

Gall bladder
(at lower end
of liver)

Large intestine

Small intestine
(not shown, in
area between
ascending and
descending
colons)

Bladder

With the right hand about one-and-one-half inches from the navel, gently press inward with the fingertips (Fig. 123). From this you can diagnose the condition of the small intestine.

Pain or hardness indicates congestion in these regions. Are the intestines expanded or contracted? Mucus and fat cause congestion or blockage in these regions. If unchecked, mucous stagnation can become cysts and tumors. About one in seven females has difficulty with menstruation and suffers from periodic discharges. If we eliminate the cause, which is excessive dairy consumption of milk, cheese, butter, other dairy products, sugar, fruit, fruit juices, and animal fats, we eliminate the congestion.

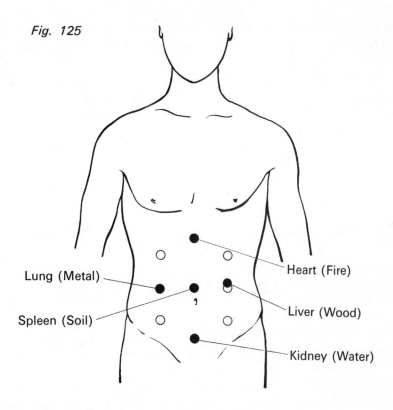

Fig. 125

Lung (Metal)

Spleen (Soil)

Heart (Fire)

Liver (Wood)

Kidney (Water)

Points 1, 2, 3, 4, and 5 are the most common locations for mucus to accumulate. Placing the hand on these points will reveal the condition of the meridian. Energy within a meridian will be either full (*jitsu*) or empty (*kyo*).

Fig. 126

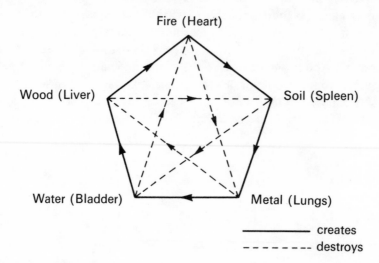

Fire (Heart)

Wood (Liver)

Soil (Spleen)

Water (Bladder)

Metal (Lungs)

———— creates

– – – – – – – destroys

The ancient practitioners of classical oriental medicine discovered a method of diagnosing the body's internal condition by feeling the *hara*. Included in this *hara* diagnosis is the Theory of the Five Transformations or Elements.

Simply stated, the stimulation of one organ also tonifies the following organ and sedates its opposite organ. For instance, by stimulating Fire (Heart), we tonify Soil (Spleen) and sedate Water (Bladder).

52.   Place the right palm on the intestines with the left palm placed directly on top of the right. Leaning your weight into the receiver's navel area, gently but deeply knead the intestines. This should take the form of a wave-like motion, pulling and pushing. The hands remain stationary on the abdomen; they do not slide about. The motion is just like kneading bread dough.

With the heel of the right hand rub the periphery of the abdomen in a clockwise direction. Do this at least three times.

53.   Pat the chest and massage the breasts.

54.   Move to the receiver's left side. Kneel between the body and the outstretched arm. Massage her left hand as you did her right hand (step 48).

55.   Massage the lower and upper arms as was done on the right side (steps 49 and 50).

56.   Adjust the arm by bending it and pulling the wrist in an outward direction. Release the arm.

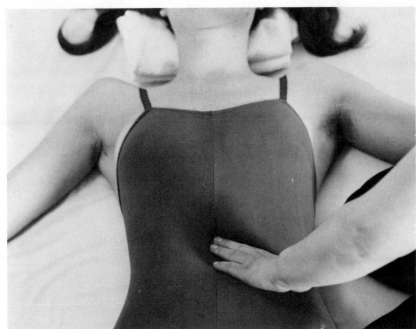

Fig. 127

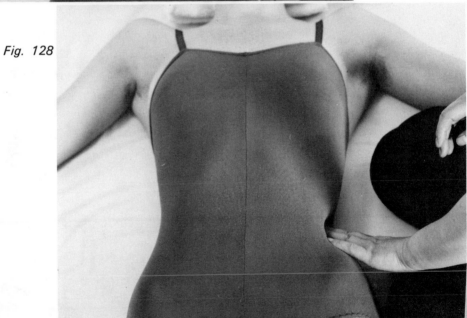

Fig. 128

57.   Check the organs located on the patient's left side. Feel the stomach. Investigate the influence of the spleen (Figs. 127 and 128). Feel

the large intestine, small intestine, and lungs (Fig. 129). Check the bladder and, in females, the ovaries and the uterus, then the pulse, which reveals the heart's activity (Fig. 130).

Knead and rub the abdominal region (Figs. 131 to 133).

Fig. 129   Fig. 130

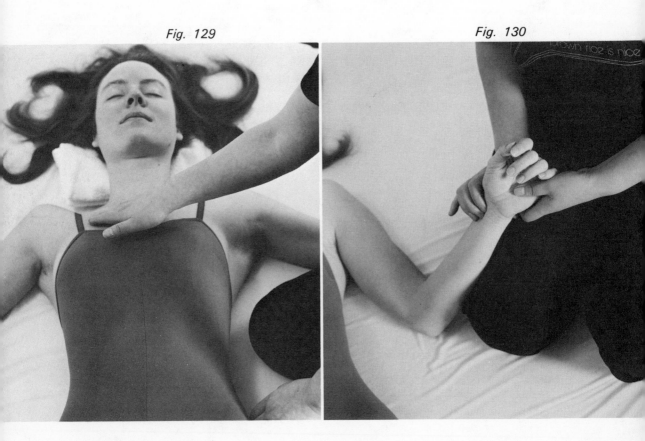

Fig. 131

Fig. 132

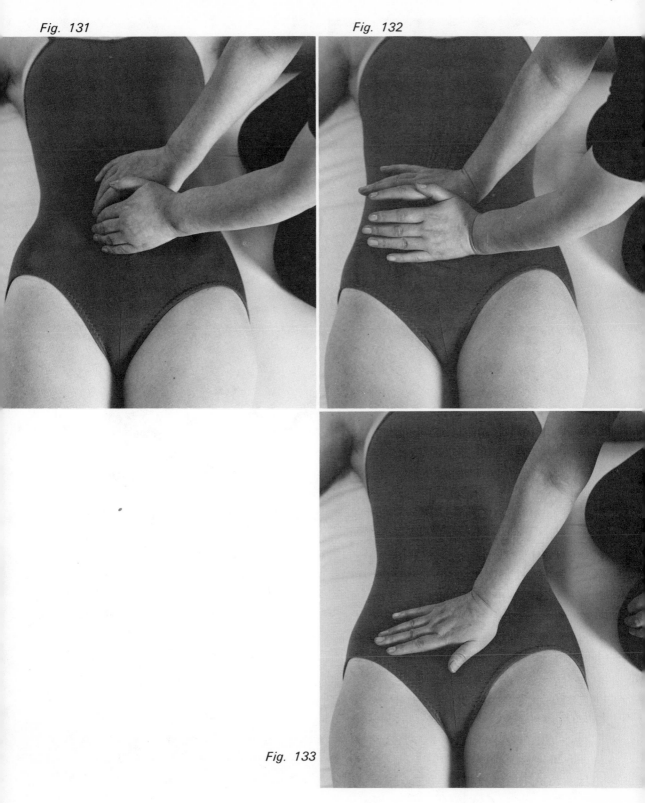

Fig. 133

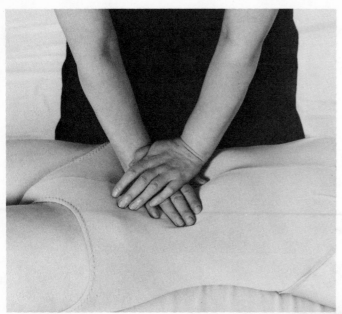

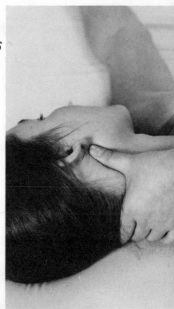

Fig. 136

Fig. 134

Fig. 135

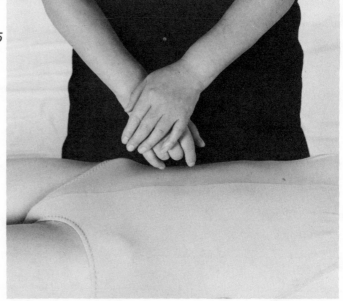

    58.   Abdominal breathing: Place your palms on the abdomen. Co-ordinate your breathing with your patient's. On exhaling, press down gently but with confidence (Fig. 134). On inhaling, lift the palms off (Fig. 135). Repeat ten times.

    59.   Place your hands behind the receiver's head (Fig. 136). You should kneel upright and face the top of the patient's head. Take several deep breaths and treat the neck.

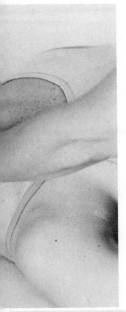

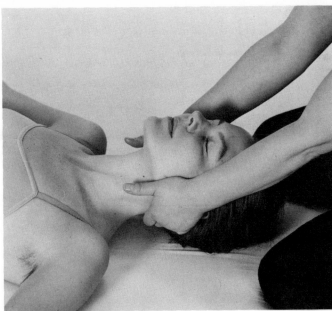

Fig. 138

Fig. 137

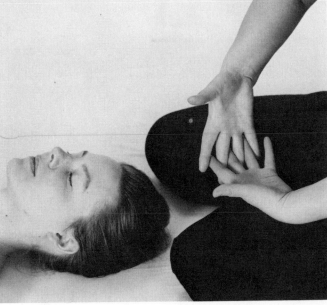

60. Kneeling behind the patient's head interlock your fingers and breathe deeply (Fig. 137). Deep, relaxed breathing calms the body and promotes concentration. Then, exhaling deeply, stretch the neck by pulling it toward yourself (Fig. 138). Push the receiver's chin on her own chest, thereby stretching the neck muscles.

Turn the neck from the center to the left side (Fig. 139). Hold it there with slight pressure. Adjust the neck if needed. While the head is turned to the left, use the right thumb to massage down the side of the neck from beneath the ear to the collarbone or clavicle.

Reverse sides and turn the head to the right side. Hold, adjust if necessary and return the head to the center.

Turn the head to the opposite side and with the left thumb massage down the left side of the receiver's neck from below the ear to the collarbone (Figs. 140 and 141).

Fig. 139   Fig. 140

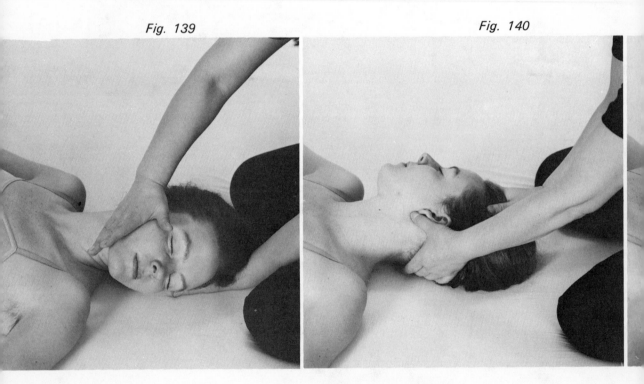

61.   With the side of your open right hand, tap the left side of the receiver's head (Fig. 142). Turn the head to the right, and with the side of your left hand tap the right side of the patient's head. There are two methods of stimulating the head, with the side of the hand and with the bottom of the fist (Figs. 143 and 144).

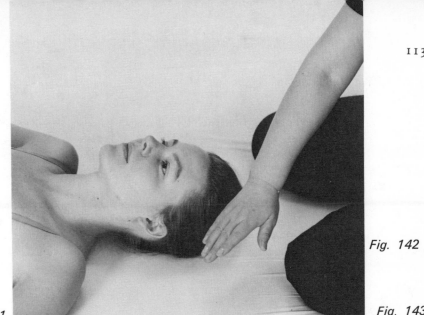

Fig. 142

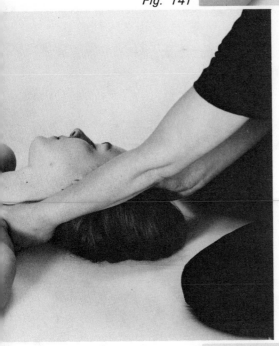

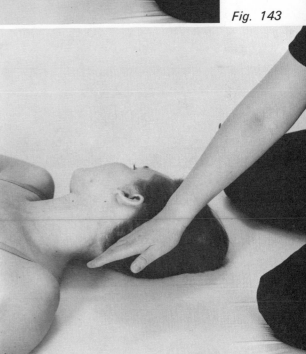

Fig. 141

Fig. 143

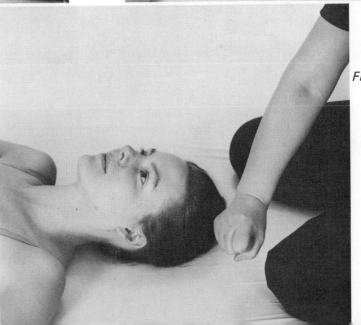

Fig. 144

62. With the thumbs together press the bladder meridians which run from the inside corners of the receiver's eyes up the forehead and down the center of the skull. Hold each point for three to five seconds. Do this three times.

Use thumb and finger pressure to stimulate the facial areas—forehead and eyes which represent the bladder and liver (Figs. 146 and 147), contours of the eyes (Fig. 148), sinus (Fig. 149), cheeks (Fig. 150), under

Fig. 146   *Fig. 147*

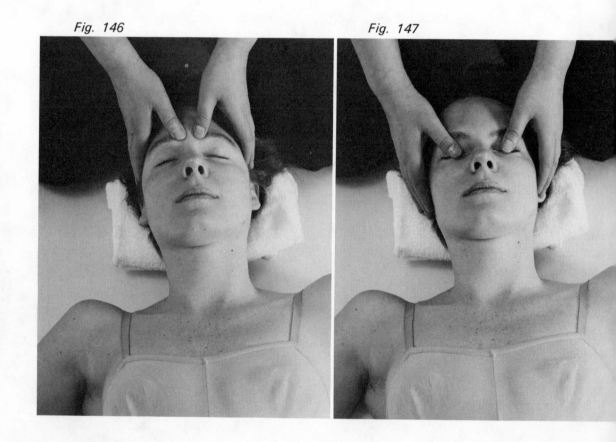

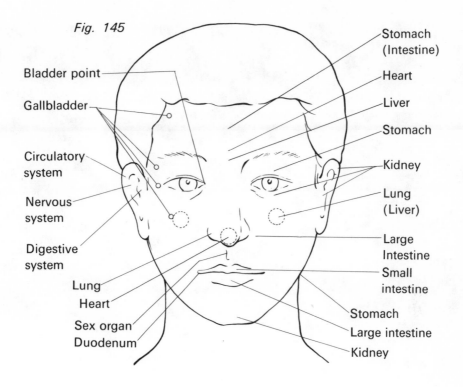

Fig. 145

Bladder point

Gallbladder

Circulatory
system

Nervous
system

Digestive
system

Lung

Heart

Sex organ

Duodenum

Stomach
(Intestine)

Heart

Liver

Stomach

Kidney

Lung
(Liver)

Large
Intestine

Small
intestine

Stomach

Large intestine

Kidney

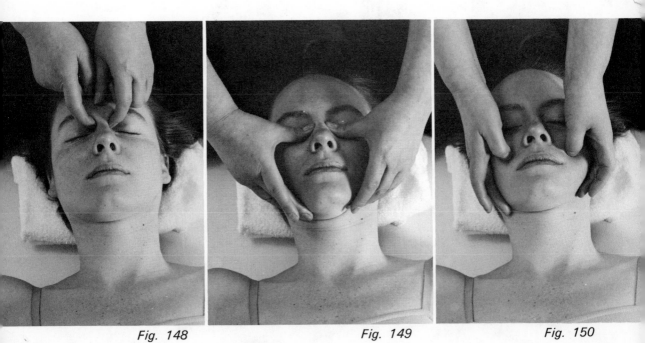

Fig. 148

Fig. 149

Fig. 150

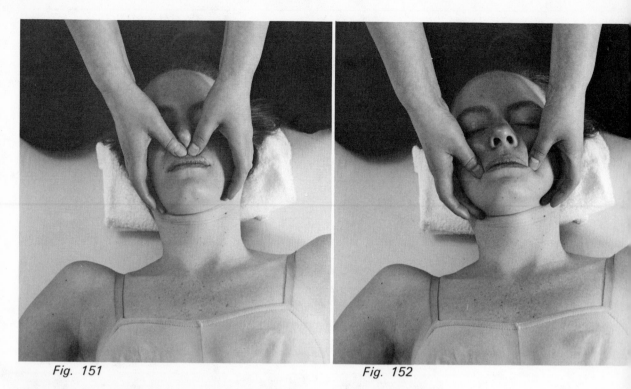

Fig. 151

Fig. 152

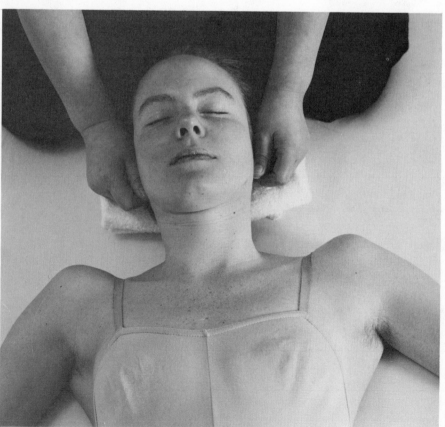

Fig. 155

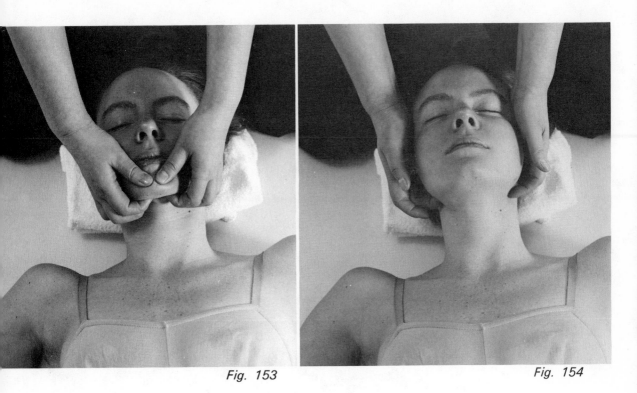

Fig. 153   Fig. 154

the nose (Fig. 151), side of the mouth (Fig. 152), chin (Fig. 153), jaw
and under the ear (Fig. 154). Finally pull the ears (Fig. 155).

Return to and press the temples.

It was recorded more than 4,500 years ago in *The Yellow Emperor's
Classic of Internal Medicine* that the ear is the place where all the chan-
nels meet. When there is a change in the internal organs or other parts
of the body, certain manifestations may appear in various portions of
the ear such as tenderness, structural change, or discoloration. Simply
stated, the ear represents the entire body. It shows our past and present
conditions. Stimulation to the ear can effect a change in the entire body.
Among acupuncturists, auriculotherapy, or the practice of working on
the ear, is becoming more and more popular.

Fig. 156

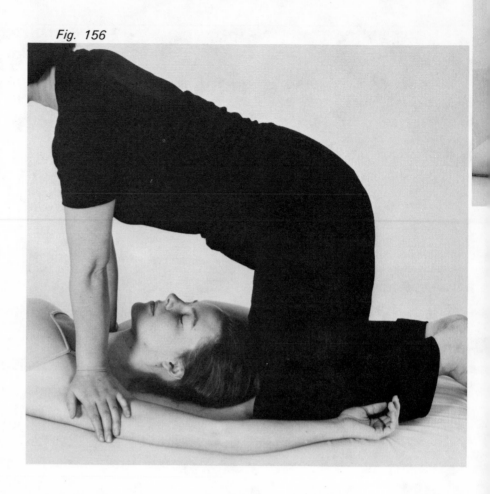

63. Holding both of the receiver's wrists, bring the arms over the head. Massage the underarm area and press (Fig. 156).

Pull the receiver's arms over her head while she pushes his heels out, thereby stretching the calf muscles (Fig. 157). This is a very good overall body stretch.

With the arms outstretched lean your body weight on the receiver's shoulders and press straight down (Fig. 158).

Massaging the inside of the arm is very good for heart troubles (Fig. 159). Press each shoulder alternately several times. Allow the patient's arms to return to a resting position at the side. Push down on the shoulders.

Experience has proven that, if possible, it is best to allow the receiver to rest for some minutes after a full session. This allows the body's energy to circulate freely, thereby effecting a change in the overall condition.

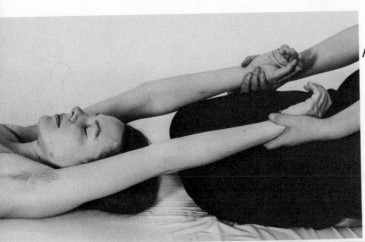

Fig. 157

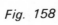

Fig. 158

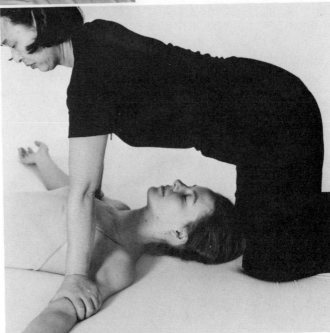

Fig. 159

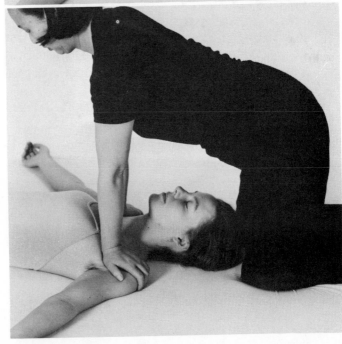

At the very beginning of our shiatsu session we observe the receiver's condition. From front, back, and side views, we begin to diagnose the overall picture of the person about to be treated. This diagnostic information determines the type and length of treatment. In short, it tells the giver, in a general way, just what is the problem. The giver then proceeds with the treatment. However, the responsibility of a cure actually rests with the receiver. The giver only stimulates and directs energy to the areas that are lacking vitality and redirects excessive energy to areas that are deficient.

After the barefoot shiatsu session, how can the receiver take responsibility for correcting the areas of his body that are in need of adjustment? Very simply, he can change the condition by consistently practicing a series of corrective exercises. Our unnatural sitting positions and bad body posture cause unnecessary stress on the body. Corrective exercises remove the sources of this stress. When posture is corrected, sickness naturally disappears. As it took time to develop the bad habits, it will take time to unlearn and correct them.

It should be understood that there are many stages in regaining health. At first there may be rapid improvement. Usually this is followed by a period of stability, but not yet complete freedom from the symptoms. For a while it may seem as though no further changes are taking place. Please remember that everything in the universe changes. The gaining of health is a step-by-step process. Changes are always going on. A seed planted in the earth needs nourishment, care and time to develop. If you realize this you will become patient. You can assure the patient that improvement will come as the situation permits. Above all, he should not worry!

If you take a relaxed attitude about your condition you will make the greatest progress. You can allow your instinctive nature to guide you in corrective exercises. For example, if the back of the neck is stiff and sore—an expanded condition—you instinctively do an exercise that will bring balance, deeply massaging or rubbing the area, thus causing contraction. Nature always strives for harmony and balance. Such harmony is regained and maintained when we receive all that nature gives us with gratitude.

Corrective exercises can be done either as homework or together with the patient during treatment.

4. Correcting Exercises

Tension in the Back

Many people have stiff spines. If you feel a person needs more stretching of the spine do this exercise.

Ask the person to lie down on the left side with arm under head. Sit at the center of the person's back. Hold opposite arms and legs; with your left hand hold the right wrist and with the right hand hold the left ankle. Put your foot in the middle of the spine (Fig. 160). The receiver's face should be turned upward. Lean backward and pull the wrist and

Fig. 160

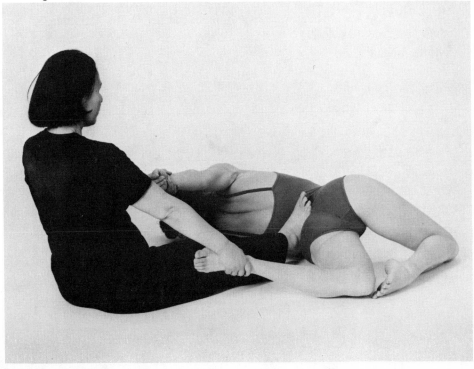

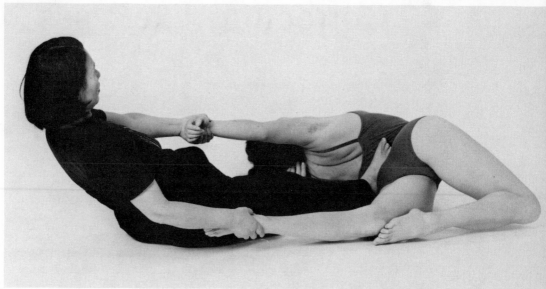

Fig. 161

ankle toward you, like a bow and arrow (Fig. 161). Coordinate your
breathing with her. Move up the spine from the hip to the shoulder
blade, one breath to each stretch. Have the receiver turn over and work
on the other side.

Fig. 164

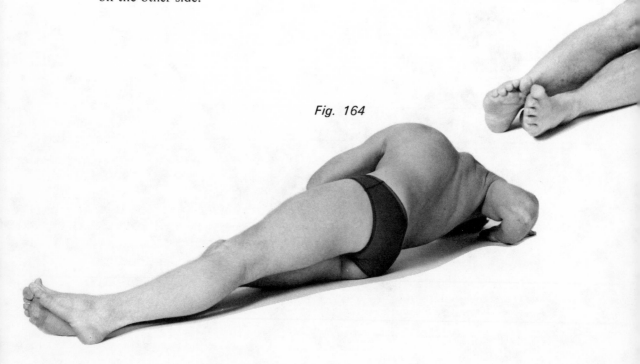

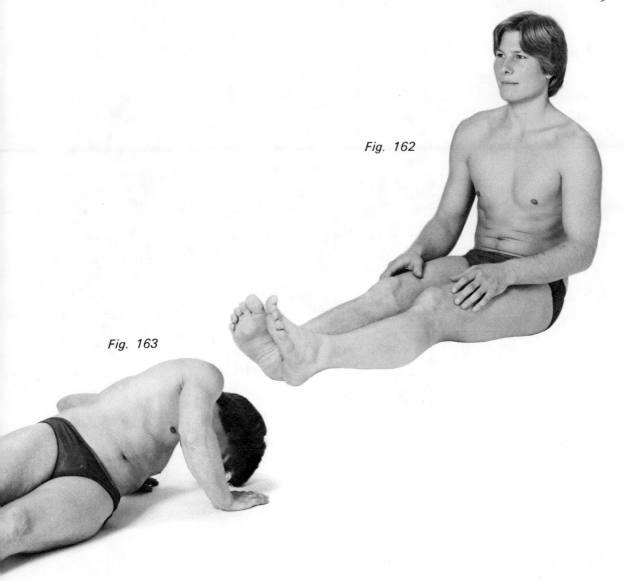

Fig. 162

Fig. 163

Twisted Spine

This exercise has a beneficial effect on the hips and helps to correct the spine.

Ask the person to sit on the floor and stretch out the knees (Fig. 162). Put one hand, and then the other, behind the back on the floor and bend the body backward (Fig. 163). Touch the head on the floor. Turn over and work on the other side (Fig. 164). If the legs are closed the upper part of the spine will be stimulated. If the legs are open the lower spine is stimulated.

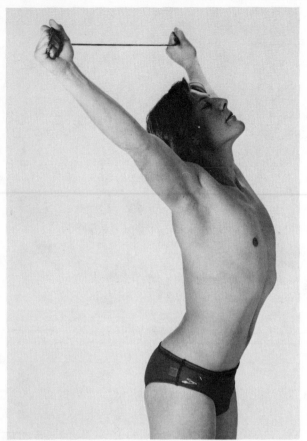

Fig. 165

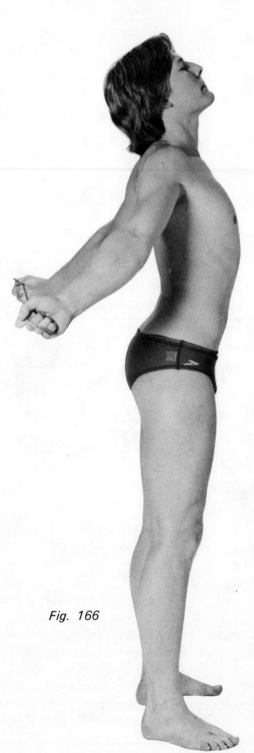

Fig. 166

Rounded Back

Recommend that the person use a rope or stick to stretch the center of the back (Figs. 165 and 166). Exercise 4 is also helpful for this problem.

Tension Between the Shoulder Blades

Ask the patient to sit or stand with the palms outstretched and facing upward (Fig. 167). The receiver should inhale and hold her breath. Bending the arms, pull the elbows back as the patient holds the face up and the chest out (Fig. 168). Ask the patient to tense the area between the shoulder blades completely. Ask her to release 90 percent of her breath and then suddenly relax. Repeat this exercise several times. The yoga *asana* called the fish pose is also very good for releasing tension in this area (Fig. 169).

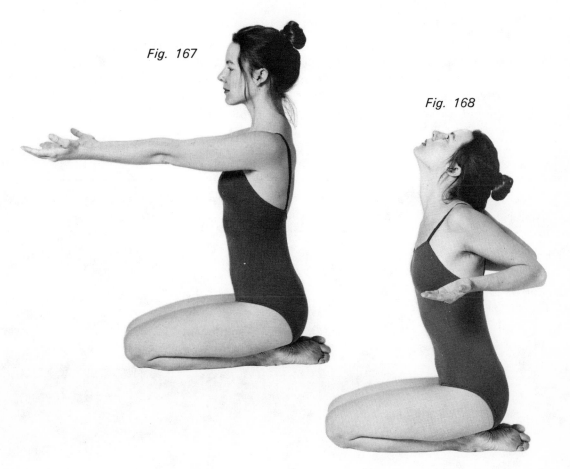

Fig. 167

Fig. 168

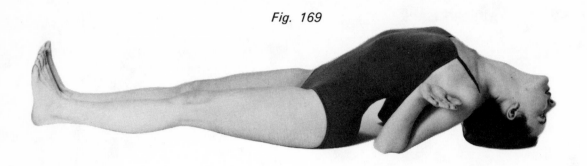

Fig. 169

Body Imbalance

Many people have balance difficulties. The balance may be shifted to either the left or the right side of their bodies. For example, if someone is standing with the right foot slightly behind the left, this means that the balance is toward the right side. The person favors the right, showing that there is trouble on this side of the body.

Ask the receiver to lie down with the toes pointed upward and the heels pushed out. Place the overactive side (left in this case) over the underactive foot. Ask the receiver to raise the legs off the floor one or two inches, making an up and down movement and then a side-to-side movement several times (Fig. 170). This is performed on the exhalation phase of the breath. This exercise balances both sides of the body.

Fig. 170

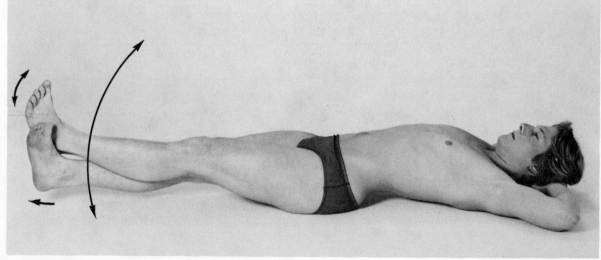

Fig. 171

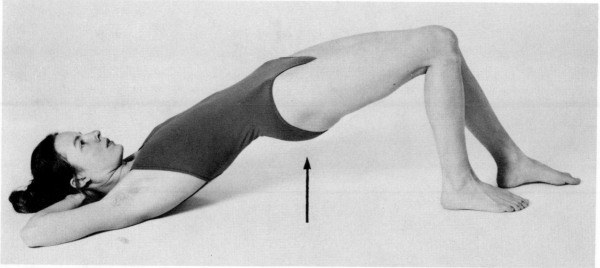

Fig. 172

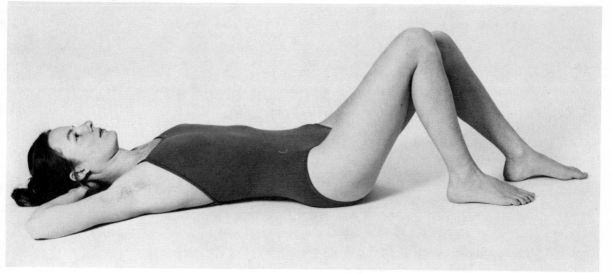

Tilted Hipbone

To correct uneven hips ask the patient to lie down on her back and bend her knees so that the feet rest near the buttocks. Place the foot that is on the side of the lower hip nearer the buttock—if the right hip is lower, place the right foot closer to the buttock. Raise and lower the back, inhaling on the up movement and exhaling on the down movement (Figs. 171 and 172). Repeat several times.

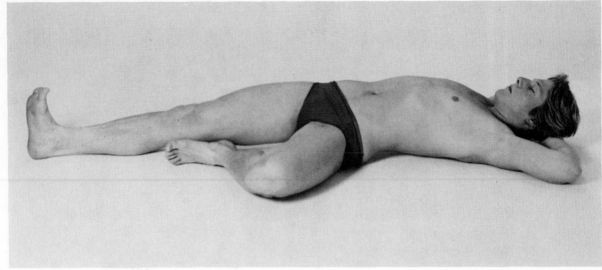

Fig. 173

Unbalanced Hip and Contracted Sides

If the receiver lies on his back you can see whether one leg is longer than the other. The shorter leg shows which side of the body is contracted. Permit the leg on the side of the contraction to remain outstretched, with heel out and toes in—a contracted right side has the right leg outstretched. Bend the opposite leg at the knee and bring the sole of the foot to the inside of the other knee (Fig. 173). Ask the patient to inhale and hold his breath. On exhalation, he must bend and stretch the upper body away from the contracted side (Fig. 174). After 90 percent exhalation, relax. Do this several times.

Uneven Shoulders

Ask the receiver to lie on her stomach, with her hands to her sides. Place the lower shoulder forward in order to make the shoulders even (Fig. 175). In this position have her perform the *cobra asana*: inhale, hold the breath, then slowly lift the head and the chest on exhalation.

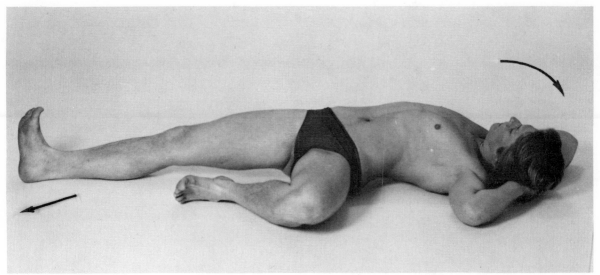

Fig. 174

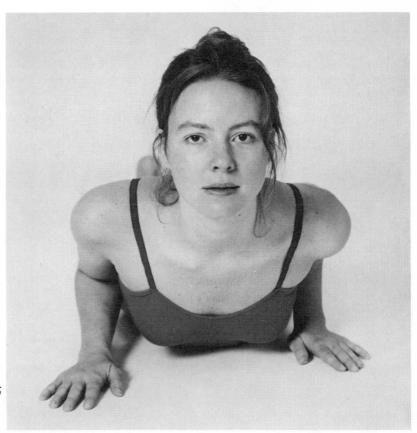

Fig. 175

130

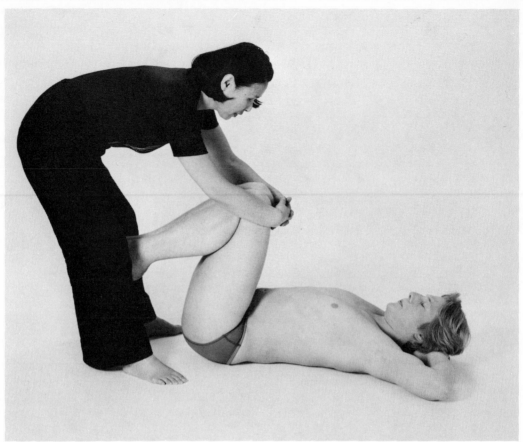

Fig. 176

Fig. 177

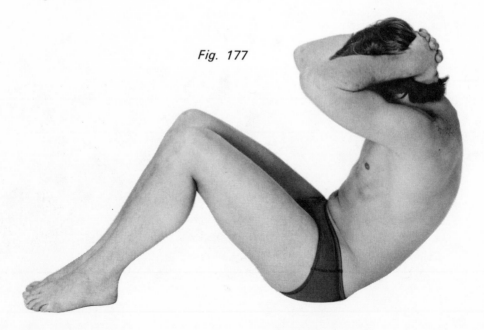

Expanded Abdomen

Many people need a strong exercise for toning the abdomen. This is
an especially good exercise for those with no power in the *hara*.

Ask the person to lie on his back with the knees bent. Hold his knees
(Fig. 176). Inhale with him and hold the breath. On exhalation, as the
receiver pulls the knees to the abdomen, the giver resists.

For homework the patient may do sit-up type exercises (Fig. 177).

Lower Back Problems

Ask the receiver to lie on his stomach. This makes the lower back contract. As the receiver bends his knees and pulls his legs forward, offer
some resistance (Fig. 178). This movement strengthens the lower back
and sexual activity.

Fig. 178

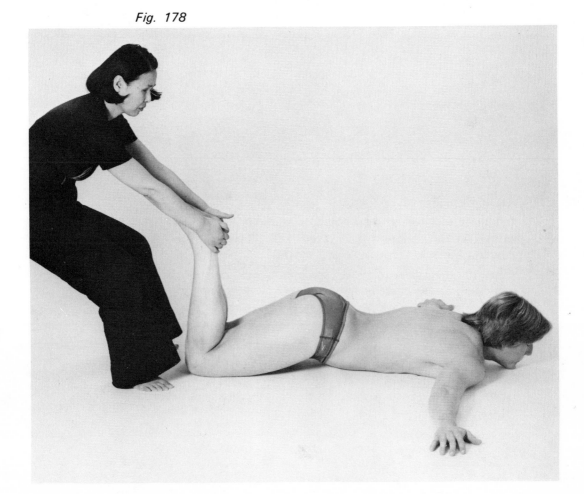

132

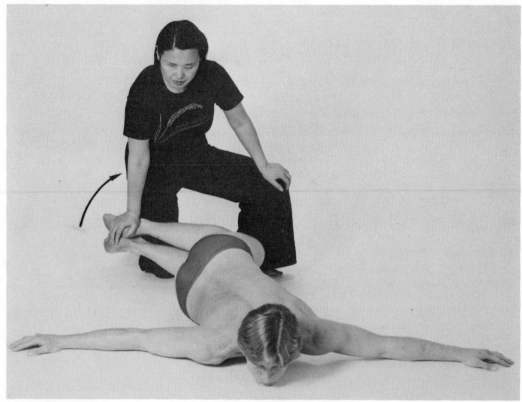

Fig. 179

Waist and Middle Back Problems

Ask the patient to lie face down. Bring the legs together, bend the knees and allow both feet to go to the floor at the side. The giver resists the receiver's effort to raise the legs (Fig. 179). This should be performed on both sides.

Ask the receiver to turn over to lie on her back. Bend the knees and bring them to the chest. Allow the knees to drop to the side. Offer resistance while the receiver tries to raise the knees (Fig. 180).

While lying on the back with knees bent, she must bring the knees together and move them from side to side (Fig. 181). This stimulates the middle organs—spleen, liver and so on—and keeps the spine supple.

With experience and observation, you will begin to see a person's balancing point. Then you can create your own balance exercises.

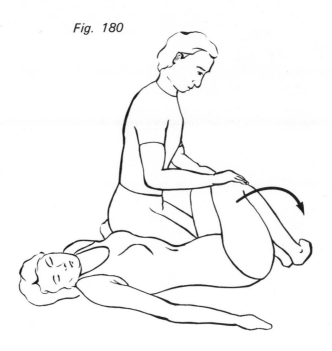

Fig. 180

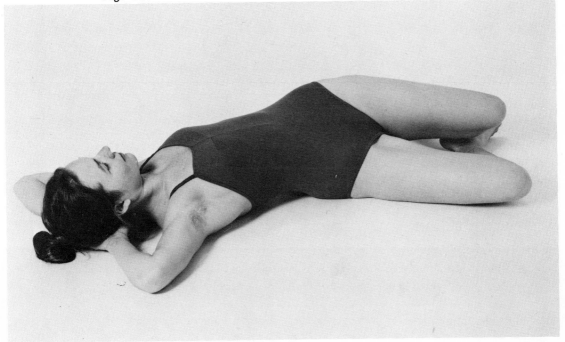

Fig. 181

5. Intuition

The chapter on training the whole person emphasizes developing the body to be sensitive and strong, and developing the mind so that its function of perception will be clear, prompt, and accurate. The techniques are consciously accomplished by will and effort. Conscious attention is given to the present condition and effort is made to improve and develop it. This valuable straightforward approach is the means used in most institutions of education.

Is there a source of information besides teachers and books? Have you thought why the foundation of a strong and healthy body and mind are necessary? Mind and body, in unity, create the condition in which another source of information is at your disposal. Having developed your abilities consciously, you are now ready to develop unconsciously. Intuition, or the quick perception of truth without conscious attention, allows shiatsu treatment to go beyond mere technique.

Instinctive knowledge about the condition of another person and the proper course of treatment to follow comes from inside one's self. Intuition is not taught in classrooms or in books. It is a faculty that an effective shiatsu practitioner must possess. Though memorizing pressure points and learning various techniques or types of pressure and manipulation are invaluable it is not information, but the touch of another human being, that stimulates the body to heal itself. If the practitioner combines technical information and proper technique and is guided by intuition, success will be achieved.

All energy comes from the infinite universe. There are seven levels through which energy passes from infinity to mankind. The Spiral of Creation shows the course of physical and material manifestation (Fig. 182). All ki (life force energy, intuition, etc.) comes from infinity and passes through various stages of physicalization. Infinity changes into positive and negative, yang and yin, which continue in an inward spiral movement toward material manifestation. From infinity, ki continuously transforms from the world of vibration, to the states of pre-atomic particles, elements, the vegetable kingdom and the animal kingdom, of which human beings are the last creation. From mankind, energy moves back outward on an expanding course, returning to one infinity.

Intuition comes from infinity. Intuition functions when resistance in

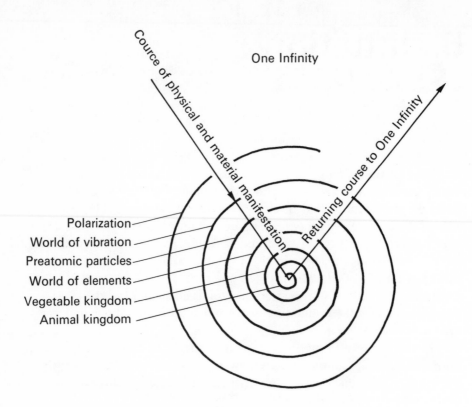

Fig. 182   Spiral of Creation

the individual is absent. Remove rigidity, which is a product of life-style, and naturally the openness necessary for intuition to flow is there. This point cannot be stressed enough. You do not need to do anything. Your investigation into your physical and psychological inflexibilities will naturally bring about the receptive state necessary for intuition to function.

Developing Confidence

At the first level of shiatsu practice, you learn various techniques and much intellectual information. You lack experience and, therefore, confidence. In order to be effective you must have confidence that you can handle any situation and respond accurately to any challenge. This assurance comes only through practice and actual work. Therefore, at first, with doubt, you must proceed to work and experience the situations that are presented to you. Reflect on these experiences. Through self-reflection and correction of your errors, assurance is gained. As you begin to trust your ability, confidence comes. When confidence is established, automatically the seeds of intuition are sown.

Unanswerable Questions

In the beginning of shiatsu practice almost all questions seem unanswerable. How much pressure can be applied to an arm, a leg, the back, the head? How long would you hold each pressure point? When is it best not to treat someone? Many of these questions have no exact answer. To the question "How much pressure am I to apply to the back?" I must answer "Who's back?" The individual condition of the receiver must always be considered. If the receiver is a hard-working male farmer the pressure most certainly will be different from that for a female senior citizen who has worked her whole life behind a desk. Generally, yang type persons have acute problems, so you can treat them with strength. Yin people, like older persons and children, need to be treated more gently.

It is the search for the answers to these unanswerable questions that is important. An exact answer will always elude us. Even the same person at different times of the year will need different pressure. This uncertainty is the challenges that stimulates development of intuition and progress in your treatment. As you learn to empty yourself of expectations and information, the answers will come quickly.

In treatment never give 100-percent effort. Generally give about 80-percent effort. This allows the person to heal himself and to accept the responsibility for his own health. With an empty mind, a centered body and 80-percent effort, seemingly unanswerable questions unfold their mysteries to you. Without attachment to achieving results, proceed with caution and confidence.

The development of a strong midbrain will allow intuition to function smoothly. The exercises in this book bring about a balanced biological condition that will stimulate the brain. As the blood quality improves, the brain will perceive more clearly.

The compact (yang) brain and nervous system receive and assimilate vibration (yin). The more expanded (yin) digestive system receives and assimilates a more dense vibration, food (yang). These two systems complement each other as receivers of external vibration, but at the same time they are antagonistic to each other. The brain receives heaven's

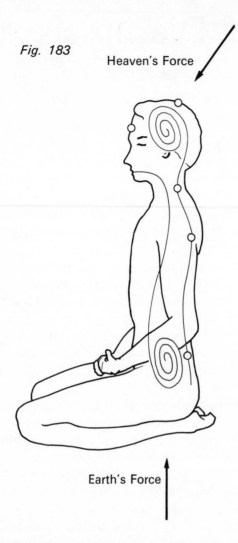

Fig. 183

Heaven's Force

Earth's Force

force (yin) and the digestive system receives earth's force (yang) (Fig. 183).

In the development of intuition both systems must function well. Any disturbance of one system will affect the harmonious performance of the other. Overeating will lessen mental clarity just as emotional problems spoil the digestive function.

To hasten intuitive development the following suggestions are recommended:

    a.   Eat little.
    b.   Be active.
    c.   Be grateful.

6. Self-Diagnosis

Just as the seasons of the year are constantly changing, so are our bodies. This fantastic movement that governs the earth and all that is on it never ceases to function. Change is continuous. For you to be in harmony with this change you too must persevere by continuing your routine of training. You cannot train your body once in a while or for a few hours here and there and expect to drive great benefit from such sporadic effort. You must train your whole body daily until the end of your life. It is very easy to go backward when you do not train.

Training should be an enjoyable part of your life. Without a deep understanding of change and of why you should train, you will be unable to continue. You will be unable to stick with the routine that you yourself have designed. Without understanding, training will be torture, and you will soon give up.

You should watch yourself carefully. Self-diagnosis enables you to be attentive to the changes that occur in your own condition. The periphery of the body, such as the hands and feet, show many symptoms very easily. The fingers and toes are either the beginning or the end of the meridians of ki flow within the body. Ki from heaven and from earth enters the body through these points. Manual stimulation of the hands and feet will help circulate this life energy.

You can observe your own hands and feet quite easily. This is why we show you this easy method of self-diagnosis. If you watch yourself and know your own condition, then you can understand another person's condition without difficulty. With observation of the parts of your body you can understand their relationship within the body. For example, if you notice something is wrong on a fingernail, you know there is trouble on the inside. Or, if you cut a finger, the place where you cut yourself relates to a weak part of your body. The accident or injury gives you a warning. Even if you just drop something, it shows that you are out of balance, either too yin or too yang. You need a mirror to see your own face, but with the hand and foot this is not necessary. We always like to do things the easy way without special equipment.

Major Observation of Self-diagnosis

The condition of all bodily systems is reflected in the quality of the three major observations of self-diagnosis. If you do not satisfy the following requirements, there is an imbalance in your life. The following is a checkup of your daily condition.

Good Bowel Movement

You should have a bowel movement at least once a day. The best condition is to have a bowel movement after each meal, as babies do. The color of the stool should be light brown to slightly dark brown. What you eat affects the color of the stool. The stool should be shaped like a banana and it should stay in one piece that floats. The odor should not be unpleasant, nor should the stool be unpleasant to look at. If your stool is very dark in color and smelly, this means that you are over-eating or taking in too much animal quality food. After the bowel movement you should have a feeling of emptiness.

Good Sleep

The definition of good sleep means the ability to lie down and go to sleep immediately. You should sleep deeply and soundly without dreaming. Then, when you awake, you will feel refreshed and ready to go on to the next activity. It is not necessary to sleep for a long time. The quality of sleep depends not on the amount of time spent in bed, but rather on how deeply you sleep. If you do not sleep this way, the physical body has a problem, such as a stiff neck or rigid hips. There may also be psychological and emotional problems. Sometimes when you overexert yourself you do not sleep well. It is much more common, however, that physical activity during the day is insufficient. Overeating and hunger also affect sleep.

Good Appetite

A person with a good appetite, one who enjoys eating good, simple foods—whole grains such as brown rice or millet, and vegetables such as onions or carrots—and who has no dislikes, can be considered healthy. Hunger that is consistent is best, as are regular eating patterns and eating about the same sized portions daily. It is not good to eat a great amount for a day or two, and then to eat nothing for a while. This erratic pattern is a sign of imbalance. One should be slightly hungry most of the time.

There are other, secondary observations that one can make to understand one's own condition.

Urine: It is normal for a human being to urinate between four and five times during the day. If you urinate more than this amount you are probably taking in excessive amounts of liquid. The urine should be the color of light beer. It should be clear, not cloudy and should not have any blood in it. Urine should flow easily. Males with prostate problems have difficulty urinating. It is painful, and the flow does not come easily.

Menstruation: Women can diagnose themselves by observing their menstrual cycle. A normal cycle is every twenty-eight days, usually at the time of the full moon. The average length of the menstrual flow should be from four to five days. There should be no pain or cramps. If the flow is longer than five days or is excessive, you are eating too much animal food. If the flow comes too early or too late, there are possible liver problems.

Hair: Females should have much less hair than males. There should be very little hair on the face, hands and legs.

There are stories about very long-lived and healthy people from various parts of the world. Just what does a healthy person look like? It is such an uncommon experience for us to find a truly healthy person that perhaps you have no idea. In Vilcabamba, Ecuador, there are people who live to be over 100 years old. The men have thick, dark hair and eye-brows, and hair sometimes comes out of their ears. This hair is very strong and resembles that used in horse brushes. Their hair resembles that of oriental peoples, but the face structure is thin, more like that of the Irish or Scots. In Ireland or Scotland, the Vilcabambans would feel at home.

The women also have a healthy head of hair which remains dark even after 100 years. The black hair color may become bluish, but not white. You can find, in women over 100 years old, long hair growing to below the hips. The women do not grow facial hair and even older women do not have moustaches. They always look very feminine.

The Vilcabambans' eyes are either blue or brown. Even in old age they retain good vision. In Europe, blue-eyed people usually lose their vision faster than brown-eyed people. In Vilcabamba, however, this is not the case. The older people have beautiful, strong eyes that shine. They look at you directly and have long, strong eyebrows and long eyelashes. The ear is especially big and long. The nose is high. The face is egg-shaped and well-proportioned. They are handsome. The people are not so tall; the average height is about five feet five inches. Remarkably, there are no overweight people in Vilcabamba. Even the older people are slim. They move very quickly, like tigers. The Vilcabambans think that a person should be so thin that when he lies down on his side, a dog should be able to pass between him and the floor.

Test Your Own Condition

Exercises for Flexibility

1. The flexibility of the body is reflected in the suppleness of the hand. Try this test. Bring your palms together as in a prayer position (Fig. 184). Can you bend your fingers at the third joint so that the fingers are perpendicular to the rest of the hand? If not, you are old before your time.

2. This test is very interesting. Bring the left hand and arm across the front of your body and reach over your right shoulder (Fig. 185). Continue reaching across the left shoulder until you hold the left ear. Very simple, I hope. Do the same with the right hand. The ability to do this exercise demonstrates your overall flexibility.

3. This test is fun to do. Sit in a Japanese-style position. Spread your knees apart and allow your buttocks to rest on the floor with the knees bent to the sides. Lower yourself backward so that the back is resting on the floor (Fig. 186). Does your back rest completely on the floor or is there a large space between you and the floor? If you cannot do this exercise, there is trouble in the intestines; you are overeating.

4. Lie on your stomach with your forehead resting on the floor. Reach back with your hands and pull your feet flat to the floor at your sides (Fig. 187). How far can you bring your feet down? This exercise demonstrates leg and knee flexibility.

Fig. 186

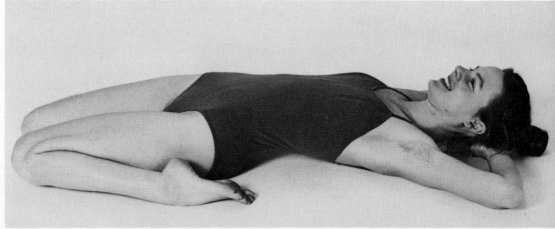

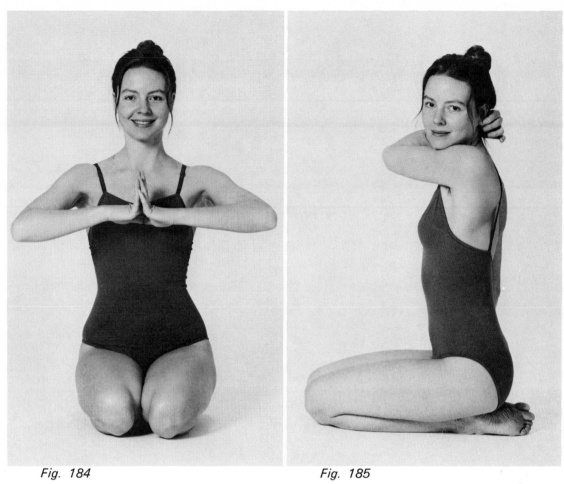

Fig. 184   Fig. 185

Fig. 187

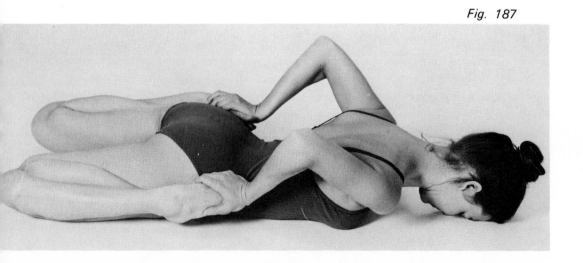

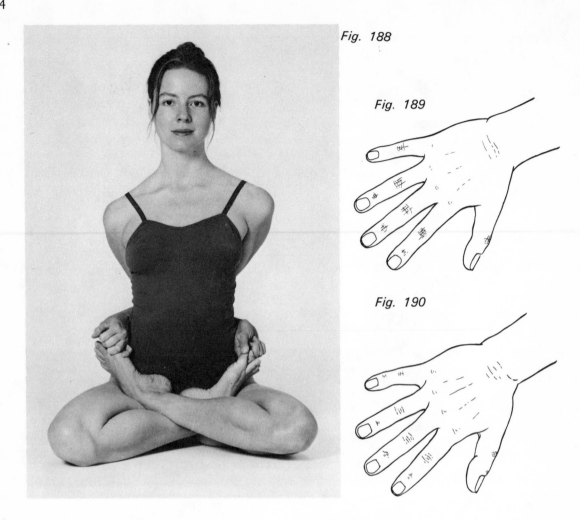

Fig. 188

Fig. 189

Fig. 190

5. If you can do this exercise, you are very flexible. Sit in lotus posture. Reach both arms behind you and, with the right hand take hold of the right toes; with the left hand, the left toes (Fig. 188).

It is very difficult to perform these flexibility exercises if you are carrying excess weight.

These five simple tests tell you about your flexibility. If there is rigidity in the body, there will be rigidity in the thinking. Self-diagnosis affords an opportunity to observe your condition so that you can actively change if you so desire. You can actually watch these changes occur.

Wrinkles in the knuckles are indicators of the digestive system's condition. A person with a properly functioning digestive system has vertical wrinkles on the center knuckles (Fig. 189). This person eats little. An overworked digestive system, because the person is overeating, has horizontal lines on the center knuckles (Fig. 190).

Yin and Yang Classification

All body types can be seen according to the theory of yin and yang. Each person is born with either a yin or yang constitution. In addition to one's constitution there is also one's present condition. You must consider these two situations when thinking about a person's condition. First consider the constitution from the parents, then consider the individual's condition. Fig. 191 very clearly demonstrates the different categories of body types. There are two yin conditions, fat and thin, and two yang conditions, fat and thin.

Fig. 191 Dietary Suggestions According to Types of Constitution

Expanded (Yin)	Contracted (Yang)
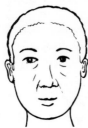	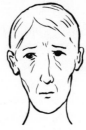
Yin and Fat Main dish: regular portion Side dish: small portion Salt: less Liquid: less Fasting: no	*Yin and Thin* Main dish: larger proportion Side dish: yang food and preparation Beverage: yang, small amount Fasting: no Keep body warm
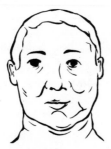	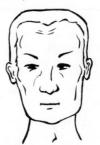

Yang and Fat
Main dish: less
Side dish: more vegetables
    (some raw)
Salt: less
Liquid: more (soup is
    recommended)
Fasting: yes
	Yang and Thin
	Main dish: soft preparation
	Side dish: regular portion
	Liquid: regular amount
	Salt: less
	Serve food warm
	Keep body warm

Dietary suggestions to improve health should suit the individual's condition and needs. A person with a yin constitution who is fat should: have a regular portion of the main dish, brown rice or another whole cereal grain; have a small portion of the side dish of cooked vegetables; use less salt and less liquid. Such people should not fast.

A person with a yin constitution who is thin should: eat a larger proportion of whole cereal grains; eat yang vegetable side dishes such as root vegetables or vegetables prepared in a yang manner—for instance, baking or long-time sautéing; drink yang beverages such as roasted green twig tea, or dandelion and grain coffees. Such people should not fast and should keep the body warm.

A person with a yang constitution who is fat should: eat less main food and more vegetables; even the addition of raw foods for a while is advisable. Such people may drink more liquid but should use less salt. Fasting is recommended.

A person with a yang constitution who is thin should: prepare the main food in a soft manner; eat a regular portion of cooked vegetables; drink a regular amount of liquid; use less salt; and serve food warm. Such people should keep the body warm.

Our physical characteristics, our tendencies, our activities, likes and dislikes, all can be seen as either yin or yang. Although this classification is very simple, there sometimes is great difficulty in accurately assessing each condition. Is your constitution and condition yin or yang? All factors should be considered. What have you done with the constitution that you have been given?

Yang (Jitsu or Full)	Yin (Kyo or Empty)
The skin is clear and smooth, neither dry nor excessively moist. It radiates life and energy. Skin color is light rose to red.	The skin is sallow, yellowish, rough, and may be excessively dry. Skin color is dark, dirty-looking. It may be pale or yellow.
The face shape is round or square. The jaw is wide. The face is fleshy.	The face shape is long and narrow. It has less flesh than average.
The eye emits strong life force. The pupil is contracted. The complexion is clear in the areas above and below the eyes.	The eye has no life force and is very weak. The pupil is expanded or very large. The areas above and below the eyes are sometimes darkly colored.

Yang (Jitsu or Full)	Yin (Kyo or Empty)
The digestive system is strong. The appetite is good.	The person has a weak digestive system. The appetite is irregular.
The bowel movement is regular, and the stool holds together. The person is prone to constipation, but a laxative brings relief.	This person goes to the toilet many times, and the stool is soft and loose. When constipated, there will be no relief even after taking a laxative.
He can take a hot bath every night and feel good.	After taking a hot bath, he feels tired.
The woman experiences regular menstruation, lasting from five to seven days. The amount of blood is excessive, and its quality is thick.	She has irregular menstruation, with a short period of thin blood.
Likes animal food, likes meat, poultry, fish, eggs, cheese, butter and salt.	Likes the sweet taste like dessert and fruit, and the sour taste like citrus and vinegar. Cannot tolerate salt.
Can drink much liquid or alcohol without great effect.	Cannot drink much or feels dull, the body swells. He loses energy and generally does not feel well.
Can eat tomato, eggplant and water-melon and feel good.	If he eats such foods, this person feels weak.
Can eat green vegetables or their juice and feels no effect.	If eaten, these vegetables cause the intestines to blow up and there is diarrhea.
Can smoke cigarettes without too much effect.	Cannot tolerate smoking.
Likes cold climates and weather.	Likes hotter climates and weather.
The voice is strong and lively. The speech is clear. There is stamina even when speaking for a long time, like lecturing.	The voice is weak and the expression is unclear. This person speaks in short sentences with many pauses.

Yang (Jitsu or Full)	*Yin (Kyo or Empty)*
The person does not sleep much and recovers from fatigue quickly.	The person sleeps many hours and still is tired. He does not recover from fatigue quickly.
The abdomen is resilient, somewhat thick and bouncing. Above and below the navel is evenly warm. The navel is deeply indented.	The abdomen is flabby and lacks resiliency. There may be cold spots around the navel. The navel itself indents only slightly.
The pulse is strong, rhythmical and even.	The pulse is weak, irregular and usually slow. Sometimes the pulse cannot be felt.
The nature is positive and aggressive. This person is very active, works hard and recovers easily.	The nature is pessimistic. This person tires very easily and has a poor recovery rate.
The movement is quick, the reactions are fast due to a strong autonomic nervous system.	This person moves and reacts slowly because the autonomic nervous system does not function smoothly.
If this person takes drugs, such as aspirin, antibiotics, and so on, there is not much harmful reaction in the digestive system.	If taking drugs, there will be a very strong reaction. Sometimes the condition gets worse and damage is done to the digestive system.
As this person grows older, the hair will turn white.	With age, this person will go bald.
The facial features are small in size and are located toward the center of the face.	The facial features are larger. The eyes are rounder, and are located toward the periphery.

Hand Diagnosis

What is a good hand? In a healthy person the hand and the face have the same pinkish coloration. The hand is clear and the color is consistent over the entire area. The texture is smooth, neither too soft nor too hard. The hand is slightly warm on all parts. If some fingers are cold or stiff, it reflects the condition of some internal organs. Each finger has flexibility.

The hand is related to the brain, therefore the quality of the emotions and the will can be seen in the hand. If a person is tense, this will show in the hand by its tense grabbing position.

The thumb is related to the autonomic nervous system, which controls the liquid in the body, the blood, lymph and the hormone systems. By manipulating the thumb, the circulatory system is affected. The thumb is also related to the digestive system. If the blood is clean and of good quality one has the power to make a tight fist. When the thumb is strong the nervous system functions well. If the thumb region has a bluish or greenish color caused by the appearance of the veins, this indicates constipation or worms. The thumb also reflects the speech center in the brain. If you treat the thumb, stuttering and other speech difficulties will be helped.

The index finger is related to the digestive system; the third finger, the circulatory system; the fourth finger, the nervous system, especially the optic nerve center; and the fifth finger, the reproductive system in the body, also connecting with the pulmonary system or the lungs.

Many relationships exist between the hand and the other parts of the body and between the hand and the body as a whole. If you use the thumb more than the rest of the fingers, there will be an overall relaxation in the body. On the contrary, if you use the little finger most, often there will be tension. A person with a strong thumb tends to have alkaline blood. Weak-thumbed persons tend to have acid blood.

Nervous disorders are reflected in stiff or shaking hands, as in the case of people prone to strokes, and in alcoholics. Use of the hands improves the memory.

People who have high blood pressure find it difficult to raise the arms completely over the head. In such cases it is necessary to manipulate the hands, neck and shoulders. The side that is most difficult to raise shows the side of the body which has difficulties. Someone who is prone to constipation usually has a stiffer right hand. People with hemorrhoids lack flexibility in the left hand.

If the wrists are stiff, this often means myopia or near-sightedness. Poor rotation ability in the wrists indicates trouble in the sex organs, bladder, kidney, and the urogenital system. A person with weak wrists often experiences hip pain. The wrists are also connected with the lungs and intestines.

In acupuncture it is noted that each finger is either the beginning or the terminus of a meridian. These meridians, or pathways of energy, pass along each finger and refer to internal organs or functions.

Along the thumb flows the lung meridian; along the index finger, the large intestine meridian; within the middle finger, the heart governor meridian which regulates circulation; along the ring finger, the triple-heater meridian, which regulates body metabolism; along the inside of the little finger, the heart meridian; and along the outside, the small intestine meridian (Fig. 192).

Fig. 192   Hand Diagnosis

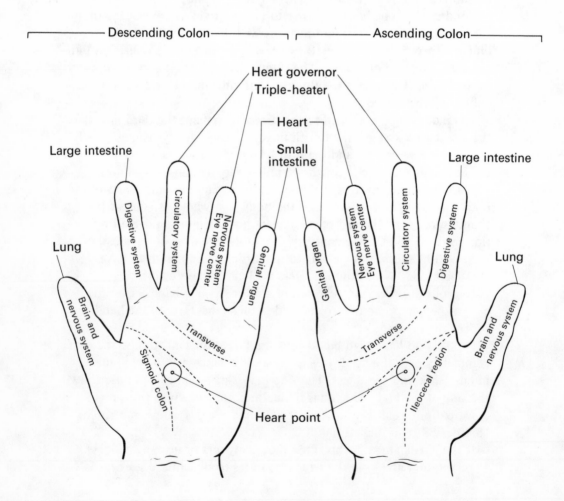

Fingernail Diagnosis

What is a healthy fingernail? The fingernails grow rather quickly: nails take from three months for a child to eight months for an older adult to change completely. The quality of nourishment is reflected in the nails. From observation of the fingernails, one can discern the condition of the person's health, especially the condition of the liver. The nail should be neither too large nor too small, neither brittle nor soft, neither too wide nor too narrow. It should be pinkish. It should not be more than one half the size of the third joint of the finger. It should be resilient and smooth, with no ridges or spots.

There are various nail shapes. (See Fig. 193.)

Fig. 193 Fingernail Diagnosis

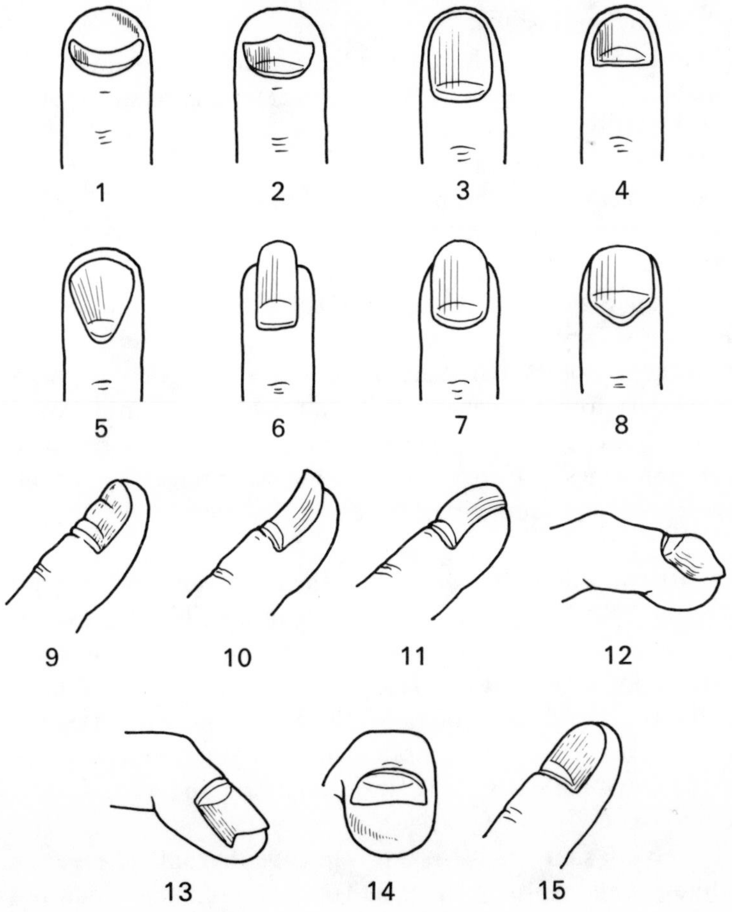

1. The very short, withered nail indicates hyperactive sensory nerves and malnutrition. This is a degenerative condition.

2. A nail that is too wide suggests hypoactive sensory nerves and dullness.

3. A person with a long nail tends to have lung and chest problems.

4. A person with short nails tends to suffer from heart problems and nervous tension and is prone to have nervous breakdowns.

5. The triangle-shaped nail shows a tendency to central nervous system problems, such as palsy or paralysis.

6. The constitution of people with narrow nails is not strong, but they have a strong will to continue.

7. An olive-shaped nail shows that the arterial system is weak. This person develops spinal trouble easily.

8. Fan-shaped nails indicate a tendency toward such liver problems as jaundice.

9. Ridges in the center of the nail indicate round worms.

10. When the end of the nail curves up, this indicates such long worms as hook worms.

11. Horizontal ridges show a condition deficient in calcium. This shape also reflects changes in situation—dietary changes or movement to another part of the country.

12. If all ten fingernails display a convex shape, a curving outward, there are problems in the bronchi such as tuberculosis or pleurisy. If the ridge is very high, there is liver trouble, arteriosclerosis, and proneness to cancer.

12. If from a side view the edges of the nail are square rather than rounded, the kidney does not function well.

14. If the top of the nail is flat instead of round, the lymph system is weak. It is easy for such persons to have mumps and tonsil troubles.

15. The presence of many perpendicular ridges shows several conditions: the intestines lack strength; the skin and circulatory system are not functioning well; sometimes the condition is acid.

There are still other ways of relating the appearance of the fingernail with internal body conditions. A person with high blood pressure has a very large moon. A big moon on the thumb nail of a person who has had a stroke indicates that the stroke was caused by cerebral hemorrhage. In a person who lacks moons, the stroke was caused by paralysis.

Very soft nails mean lack of both stamina and calcium. A person with very hard, brittle nails have an anemic condition and an unbalanced hormone system.

A person with shiny nails has an overactive thyroid, whereas someone with white-colored nails has anemia. Too much red color indicates heart problems. If they are a dark color, the circulatory system is not functioning well. A different color in each fingernail means vein problems.

White spots on the nail generally indicate too much sugar, as well as a lack of calcium. Sometimes they show the presence of worms.

Foot Diagnosis

What is a good foot? Have you ever thought of the reason why human beings are able to stand? We have been standing upright for a long time and it seems very natural, doesn't it? We stand because the first toe is very well developed. If the big toe is developed, the second toe will be able to stay close to the first one. The body's weight can be placed on the balls of the feet. It is this union of the first and second toes that forms the rounded section of the foot on which balance relies. If the first toe is developed then the Achilles' tendon can be stretched, thereby allowing one to put weight under the ball of the foot.

Proper balance is distributed in six parts. The heel receives three parts of the weight. Two parts go to the fourth toe, the last part goes under the big toe. With this distribution, the weight will go straight down to the arch. A person lacking an arch is weak because his physical constitution is weak.

Body posture and health result from the condition of the feet, hips, and spine; the distribution of body weight; and balance. For this reason, we are concerned with exercises that readjust misaligned parts of the body. The interaction of these parts make up the whole person. We realize that a problem in one area always affects the rest of the body.

The lower back region, just above the hips, is very important to correct body posture. The second lumbar vertebra controls the movement and organ functions of the lower body. The third supports the upper body weight. The fourth orders the second and the third, also controlling the hips and the rib cage. Therefore, the second, third, and fourth lumbar vertebrae form the center for all the central body movement.

The legs hold the body weight in balance. The abdomen keeps the posture in order. The brain controls both of these processes in an antagonistic-complementary manner.

If the legs are weak, there will be trouble in the hips. The upper portion of the body will be unable to maintain good posture. The legs are not only for walking or for keeping the posture erect, they aid in the circulatory function. As the legs move, blood is pumped against the force of gravity back to the heart. Weak legs contribute to a weak heart.

If the body's weight tends to fall forward, the hip will counterbalance this tendency, causing trouble in the hip area. Many women have uterus problems for this reason. If the weight is on the heel, the abdomen has no power; the back bends, and the shoulders roll forward. This condition tires one easily.

A healthy person's toes are straight and touch each other. The big toe is related to the liver and corresponds to the throat, tongue, nose, and eyeballs. If the big toe is well-developed, the person will have a very good appetite, which can sometimes lead to overeating. There may be a tendency toward diabetes or sinus congestion.

The second and third toes relate to the bronchi, the temples, the top of the head, the lips, the digestive system and the stomach.

The fourth toe relates to the gallbladder and the lungs. If this toe looks weak or bends, the person has a tendency toward lung problems such as tuberculosis. A stiff fourth toe indicates gallbladder problems and constipation.

The fifth, or little toe is related to the uterus, bladder, anus, ears, eyes, and throat. If this toe is stiff and turns downward the internal organs may be dropped or the uterus twisted. One way to make the toes strong is to use them to pick up objects.

Did you know that feet become larger as the day progresses? Feet are usually about 10 percent larger at night than they are in the morning. If a person's feet swell more than this, there are problems in the kidneys.

The old saying, "A cool head and warm feet are sure signs of health," has a lot of truth in it. When the head is cool, judgment is clear, accurate decisions can be made promptly. An overly warm head is caused by an excess of blood in the head region. This excess disrupts the thinking process and irritates the individual. Have you ever met a hothead? You very easily see the difference between the cool, level-headed person and the easily excitable hothead.

When the feet are warm, circulation in the lower region is good. If the circulation is bad in the feet and legs, the veins cannot return the blood to the heart and varicose veins may develop. In addition, the internal organs are affected and arthritis and rheumatism may develop.

Sole of the Foot

The sole of the foot is always in contact with the earth. Its condition tells us many things about the total condition of the person. The antagonistic-complementary system that exists in the body is perhaps most evident in the foot. Besides indicating bodily condition, the sole can be massaged to remedy many ailments.

A sole that is too soft means the body is undeveloped. The texture of the skin on the sole should be smooth and even. If one side of the foot is hard and the other side is soft, the upper body may be twisted. Cold

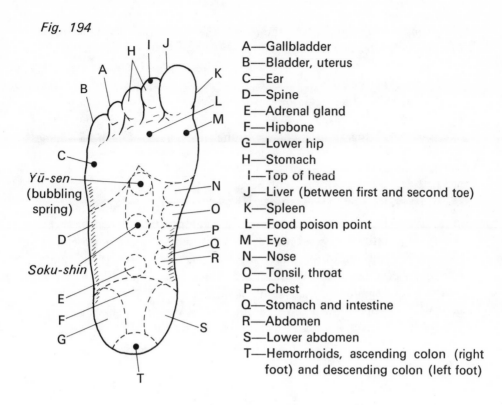

Fig. 194

A—Gallbladder
B—Bladder, uterus
C—Ear
D—Spine
E—Adrenal gland
F—Hipbone
G—Lower hip
H—Stomach
I—Top of head
J—Liver (between first and second toe)
K—Spleen
L—Food poison point
M—Eye
N—Nose
O—Tonsil, throat
P—Chest
Q—Stomach and intestine
R—Abdomen
S—Lower abdomen
T—Hemorrhoids, ascending colon (right foot) and descending colon (left foot)

feet indicate poor circulation. If the feet are always very hot, the person is prone to such skin disease as fungus. Hardening of the arteries is first visible on the feet. The sole is related to the kidneys. The arch is especially related to the throat and compresses (especially mustard) should be applied to the foot for sore throat and tonsil trouble. Massaging and pressing the sole of the foot is very beneficial in cases of drowning and fainting. Press the sole for a tired brain or for spinal problems.

Weight Distribution

If the body weight is carried on the outside of the foot instead of on the center, the anus remains open and the hip muscles cannot contract. In this situation, circulation is poor and hemorrhoids develop easily. Press the soles with a rolling pin for overall stimulation.

If the Achilles' tendon contracts and shrinks, the balance tends toward the back. This forces the abdomen into an awkward position and organs, especially the stomach, may drop. This is a cause of irregular menstruation and heart troubles.

If too much weight is placed on the heel, the ankles become weak. This in turn affects the intestines. The calves become stiff, indicating that the digestive system is weak.

It is interesting to note that the foot is the first part of the body to become cold after death.

Meridians on the Foot

All meridians either begin or end in the hands or feet. As with the hand, there are individual pathways following each toe. With manipulation we can bring about a change in the functioning of each meridian system.

The outside of the big toe relates to the spleen meridian, while the inside of the big toe relates to the liver meridian. The second and third toes relate to the stomach meridian; the fourth, the gallbladder meridian; and the little toe, the bladder meridian (Fig. 195).

The information provided here should be used as an aid in observing the overall condition of the individual. No one symptom is the ultimate barometer of a condition. We must see things as a whole. Although useful, the foregoing analysis is only a small part of seeing the whole person. Therefore, always allow common sense and intelligence to guide you in the observation and application of diagnosis.

Fig. 195

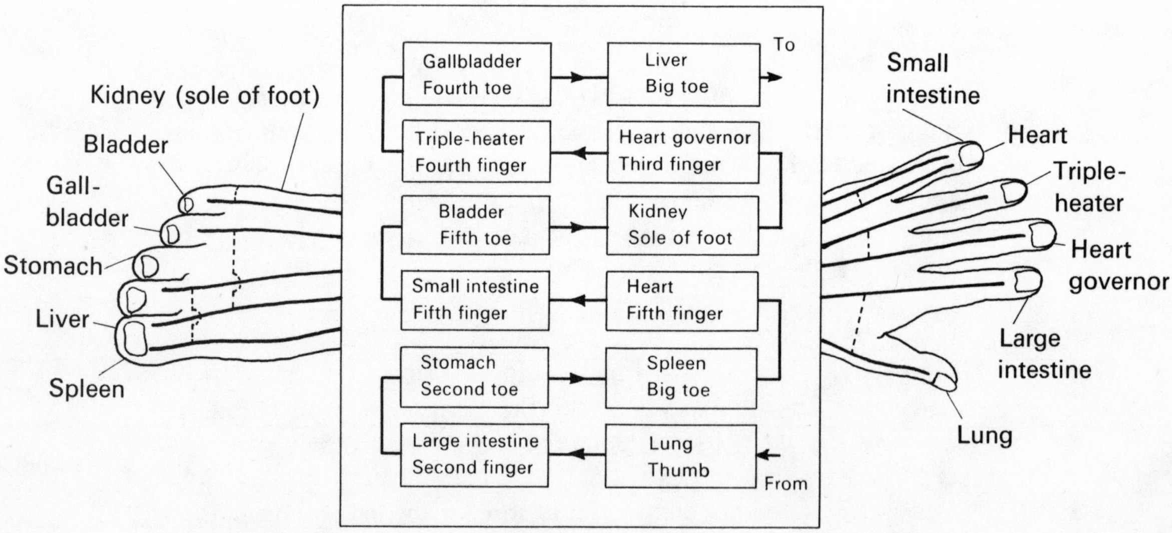

A continuous flow of energy passes from one meridian system to the next. Beginning with the lung meridian, energy passes to the large intestine meridian. From there it continues on to the stomach meridian. Eventually, it will pass through each part of the body and then begin to flow again within the lung meridian.

Conclusion

In the United States and throughout the world, rapid changes are taking place in all phases of life. Modern technologies and material achievements are revolutionizing our life-styles. This technological trend toward greater production and efficiency can beneficially alleviate many of the world's problems. On the other hand, rapid transformation in life-style today is leading toward depersonalization, and is creating significant degeneration and disintegration. The basic unit of society, the family, is being destroyed. The number of separations and divorces is astounding.

The current problems of living in the twentieth century are often felt to be so far advanced that nothing can be done to remedy their destructive course. Doomsday prophecies are easy to comprehend as we feel with all our senses that this current trend can only lead us to extermination.

One of the least developed qualities of mankind is honest, or accurate, communication. It is my hope that shiatsu can act as a bridge in unifying the communication gap, especially the one existing in the family. Honest communication using shiatsu puts families and friends in touch with each other. This can transform the family from a state of disintegration and separation to one of understanding and reunion.

Please give many shiatsu treatments to family and friends. In this way you can actively transform the world. When someone receives a good shiatsu treatment, his body and mental outlook are improved. His pessimism is changed into a general feeling of well-being. Within two years you can treat fifty people. In two more years 10 percent of those fifty people can treat another fifty persons. Within four years, 250 people are changed; and in two more years there will be 1,250 persons who have experienced the transforming energy of the healing touch through shiatsu. This increase comes if only 10 percent of those treated continue with occasional shiatsu treatments.

Please continue this practice. Movement starts with one step and grows; we plant one seed, and nature gives us many grains and vegetables in return. If you continue giving treatments, families will become closer; and all mankind will begin to be like one family. We can have a very pleasant world. I would be very happy if we all would do this.

Index